The Mindful Way through Anxiety

BREAK FREE FROM CHRONIC WORRY AND RECLAIM YOUR LIFE

Susan M. Orsillo, PhD

Lizabeth Roemer, PhD

Foreword by Zindel V. Segal

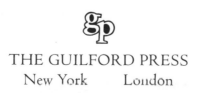

THE GUILFORD PRESS

New York   London

The information in this volume is not intended as a substitute for consultation with healthcare professionals. Each individual's health concerns should be evaluated by a qualified professional.

Printed in the United States of America

This book is printed on acid-free paper.

Last digit is print number: 9 8 7 6 5 4 3 2 1

Library of Congress Cataloging-in-Publication Data

Orsillo, Susan M., 1964–
      The mindful way through anxiety : break free from chronic worry and reclaim
your life / by Susan M. Orsillo and Lizabeth Roemer. — 1st ed.
            p.   cm.
      Includes bibliographical references and index.
      ISBN 978-1-60623-464-8 (pbk. : alk. paper) — ISBN 978-1-60623-982-7
(hardcover : alk. paper)
      1. Anxiety—Popular works.   I. Roemer, Lizabeth, 1967–   II. Title.
      BF575.A6O77 2011
      152.4′6—dc22
                                                                                    2010039235

Praise for
the mindful way through anxiety

"Potentially of great benefit to anyone suffering from anxiety in this era of relentless drivenness, social isolation, stress, and perpetual digital distraction. The authors' wise counsel based on their own clinical experience and research, coupled with vivid stories of their own and other people's lives, provide compelling evidence for why mindfulness is so important in reclaiming your life, and effective guidance in how to go about it in meaningful and very practical ways."

—*Jon Kabat-Zinn, PhD, coauthor of* The Mindful Way through Depression

"If you're looking for a fresh way of relating to—and healing—anxiety, you'll find this book an invaluable guide. The authors bring alive the path of mindfulness in a clear and accessible way."

—*Tara Brach, PhD, author of* Radical Acceptance

"This book is user friendly, practical, and quite comprehensive. Readers will benefit greatly from the insights and exercises provided in these pages."

—*Sharon Salzberg, author of* Lovingkindness

"By far the most sophisticated and engaging guide I have seen on mindfulness and anxiety. This book is a gem. Two of the field's most knowledgeable and creative experts skillfully take you on a journey into the hidden corners of your anxious mind. With a seamless blend of interesting stories, state-of-the-art research, and exercises, this book leads you step by step toward a fuller, more meaningful life. It is an excellent resource for anyone who seeks a path to freedom from anxiety and stress."

—*Christopher K. Germer, PhD, author of* The Mindful Path to Self-Compassion

"Anxiety is an emotion that begs us to mishandle it through worry and rumination. In a careful, step-by-step fashion, Drs. Orsillo and Roemer show you how to use mindfulness to break free from the grip of anxiety and move forward now toward the kind of life you want to live."

—*Steven C. Hayes, PhD, author of* Get Out of Your Mind and Into Your Life

"Whether you suffer from milder worries or a clinical disorder, this book shows you a clear, scientifically validated path toward feeling better. Lots of books propose to teach how to beat anxiety. Some are good, others less so. *The Mindful Way through Anxiety* is destined to be one of the best. Drs. Orsillo and Roemer are renowned experts in the science of beating anxiety, and their book is readable, informative, and practical."

—*David F. Tolin, PhD, coauthor of* Buried in Treasures:
Help for Compulsive Acquiring, Saving, and Hoarding

"In the Alice in Wonderland world of emotions, anxiety is the Red Queen—always a future threat and sometimes a present danger. This superb book shows how mindfulness can help ease the ravages of anxiety. Nobody knows more about this topic than Drs. Orsillo and Roemer, and their approach will be a godsend for many."

—*David H. Barlow, PhD, ABPP, Professor of Psychology and Psychiatry, Boston University, and Founder and Director Emeritus, Center for Anxiety and Related Disorders*

contents

foreword

At the turn of the 20th century, no less a psychological sage than William James recognized that the present moment offers us a wonderful vantage point from which to engage with distressing experiences. But what he was less certain of was how this could be taught to others: "the faculty of voluntarily bringing back a wandering attention, over and over again, is the very root of judgment, character, and will ... but it is easier to define this ideal than to give practical instructions for bringing it about." Things have certainly changed since then. Today, the clinical uses of meditative practices are oriented toward cultivating a particular form of awareness, known as mindfulness, which originated in the wisdom traditions of Asia. These practices, which have been taught for millennia, have been faithfully adapted for use in modern medical and mental health settings. As the authors of this wise and practical book point out, they also fit remarkably well with the needs of anxious clients who are intent on seeing beyond fitful cycles of worry and engaging with those parts of their lives inadvertently sequestered in the hope of averting further catastrophe.

Combining an accessible writing style with a surefooted clinical sense of those moments when anxiety sings its siren song of protection, the authors describe their approach with a heartfelt understanding of how difficult beginning this work can be. Going against the grain is never easy, much less for clients who are nudged to consider that many of their surefire routines aimed at reducing fear turn out to work against them. Clinical vignettes and case examples vividly illustrate how a narrow focus on the self and an unexamined preference for behaving in ways that ensure an anxiety-free life have high costs, even if they deliver relief in the short term.

The Mindful Way through Anxiety succeeds at conveying these essential insights in two distinct ways. Readers will find a gentle step-by-step structure that first educates them about anxiety in its different guises and shows the relevance of mindfulness backed by explicit guidance for developing these skills. Once established, this sturdy mental platform supports your engagement in practices that may appear at first counter-intuitive or threatening, such as befriending emotions, letting go of control agendas, or sharpening the detail of bodily sensations, but turn out to be at the core of this approach's effectiveness. In addition, Drs. Orsillo and Roemer's work follows in the best behavioral and cognitive tradition of teaching people how to change their relationship to anxiety rather than eliminate it. Chapter by chapter, the reader comes to appreciate how each of the specific interventions have embedded within them the same metamessages of awareness, investigation, and compassion.

Many readers will use this book effectively on their own, but because the format of their treatment can be so easily incorporated into the framework of individual therapy, readers may choose to work with a clinician to develop mindfulness skills in the context of regulating their emotions. As demonstrated in outcomes from numerous clinical trials, drawing on these skills throughout the day makes it easier to allow distressing moods, thoughts, and sensations to come and go without the need to battle them. In time, those willing to commit to the practice come to see that it is possible to take a wholly different approach to the endless cycles of mental strategizing that are part and parcel of anxiety disorders. What often comes as a surprise is that the route taken for this new learning leads them to discover a range of inner resources for growth and healing that they may not even have believed they possessed. What is clear is that on some occasions this new relationship with anxious thoughts and feelings can cause those feelings to abate, whereas at other times the best one can do is achieve a sort of détente with his or her problematic emotions so that even in their presence there is more room for living and valued action. Drs. Orsillo and Roemer have done both therapists and their patients a tremendous service in offering *The Mindful Way through Anxiety* as a guide to this valuable but perennially challenging process.

ZINDEL V. SEGAL, PHD, *University of Toronto*

acknowledgments

So many people have contributed to this book, by inspiring and influencing our ideas, contributing to the process and content of our approach to treating anxiety, and supporting us personally and professionally. It's a daunting task to try to acknowledge them all and we're sure we have left some important people out. Interconnections and influences of ideas and insights are so pervasive that we can't accurately identify them all. So we would like to begin by expressing our gratitude to everyone who has contributed to our work, our lives, and this book, in any way, including those who provided large and small offerings of support and encouragement (such as serving us sustaining food and providing carpooling services), those who challenge us regularly to practice and apply our skills, and, of course, those who have shaped our thinking about mindfulness and anxiety.

Still, we would like to try to name some key people who helped make this book and our work together happen. We are extremely appreciative of the pioneers in the field who showed us how cognitive-behavioral therapy could be deepened and enhanced with the integration of acceptance and mindfulness. Their work inspired a profoundly satisfying decade of personally meaningful clinical research aimed at developing and testing the ways that effective therapies might better promote life transformations. For this we thank Mark Williams, John Teasdale, Zindel Segal, and Jon Kabat-Zinn, authors of *The Mindful Way through Depression*, for modeling how to skillfully convey the healing potential of mindfulness to help people struggling with depression and for inspiring our work with anxiety. We particularly thank Zindel for his continual support of our work and our development over the years. Similarly, we are deeply grateful to Steve Hayes, Kelly Wilson, Kurt Strosahl, and Sonja Batten, whose work with acceptance and commitment therapy (ACT) has informed and influenced our work immensely over the years. Many of the exercises, metaphors, and principles in this book are drawn from ACT. We're also grateful to the many other psychologists who directly influence our work, including Andrew Christensen, Sona Dimidjian, Christopher Germer, Leslie Greenberg, Neil Jacobson, Marsha M. Linehan, Alan Marlatt, Christopher Martell, Doug Mennin, Ron Siegel, and Paul Wachtel, as well as the Buddhist writers who shape and inspire us, including Ezra Bayda, Tara Brach, Pema Chödrön, Lin Jensen, and Sharon Salzberg.

We thank Tom Borkovec and David Barlow for their pioneering work in the understanding and treatment of anxiety and worry, which forms the sturdy foundation that we attempt to build on here. In addition to the tremendous contributions both have made as scientists and scholars in the field, they have specifically informed and supported our current line of research. We are deeply grateful to Kitty Moore at The Guilford Press for encouraging us to write the book, believing we had something important to share with people, and supporting us throughout the process. We are extremely appreciative for the care and sensitivity Chris Benton brought to the task of helping us communicate our ideas clearly and effectively. This book benefited immensely from her ability to translate our intentions into easily readable prose. We also thank Paul Gordon for designing such a beautiful cover.

We are indebted to Sarah Hayes-Skelton for skillfully overseeing our grant while we were immersed in the book and, more important, for sustaining us with her friendship and support. We also thank Sarah and the other therapists we work with for sharing their wisdom and experience to help us further develop our understanding of how mindfulness can transform lives and free people from worry and anxiety. Most of all, we are grateful to the clients we and our therapists have worked with over the years. Their courage and willingness to turn toward their emotions and move toward living lives that matter to them have inspired and motivated us to share their lessons with other people struggling with anxiety.

I (S. M. O.) am truly blessed to have had the opportunity to write this book with my long-term colleague and friend, Liz. It is a rare privilege to collaborate with someone who can simultaneously inspire, challenge, and support your work in the ways that Liz has through our 15 years of shared research and scholarship. Even more rare is that this collaborative relationship is intertwined with such a deep and sustaining friendship. Thank you, Liz, for the immeasurable ways you contribute to my personal and professional life. I also had the good fortune while writing this book to be surrounded by an amazingly supportive and fun group of students and colleagues at Suffolk University. A special thanks to Lisa Coyne, Gary Fireman, Amy Marks, David Pantalone, Tracey Rogers, and Lance Swenson for their continuous support and friendship. I appreciate the close network of friends and neighbors, particularly Cathy McCarron and Kelly Bukovich, who graciously provided a watchful eye and shuttle service to my kids when I was immersed in writing. Finally, I am deeply thankful to my family for their support of my work. Thanks to my parents, for their unshakable confidence in my ability to pursue my academic goals. Also to my children, Sarah (14) and Sam (12), for being willing to genuinely invite mindfulness and valued living into our home and for allowing me to share some of their stories. Most of all, I am thankful for the steady and unfailing love, support, and encouragement of my husband, Paul. In addition to helping in every practical way to co-manage our crazy, hectic life, Paul has supported and understood my need to deeply engage in this work and to incorporate it into our shared life.

As always, I (L. R.) find myself at a loss for words when trying to express my appreciation for Sue. Our friendship and collaboration is sustaining and enriching and makes everything—this book, our research, my thinking, the dance party at our annual conference, my life—better. One of the great joys of writing this book has been the way we worked together, each one stepping in when the other was depleted for various reasons, always improving both the process and the content with our partnership. I also can't possibly find the words to capture my immense gratitude for my husband, Josh, whose wisdom, care, skillfulness, support, and experience contributed to every aspect of creating this book. Josh's deep commitment to "not sparing the dharma's assets" led to his insights being reflected throughout the book, without attribution. From the first moment we were asked to write the book, Josh's deep belief in our ability to write something that could truly be of service to others has sustained my faith in that ability and kept me writing, rewriting, revising, and revising again. He has patiently provided advice and guidance on every aspect of the book, from important ideas to vivid examples to specific word choices, always improving the work with his contributions. And his love, partnership, and friendship help me keep living a life that matters to me every day. As always, I thank my students past and present (and future) for teaching, inspiring, and motivating me and enriching our work. I'm also deeply grateful for all the friends and family, particularly my parents, who love and support me, even when I'm immersed in an all-consuming task and not nearly as attentive as I'd like to be. Thanks especially to Carolyn, whose grace and courage during a tragic time was a source of inspiration, and whose friendship is always cherished. I also thank the members of the Boundless Way Zen and O2 Yoga communities for their support and their teachings.

Finally, we thank the National Institute of Mental Health for supporting our work and this book with grants MH63208 and MH074589.

introduction

HOW THIS BOOK WILL HELP YOU

Fear and anxiety are like a pair of overzealous bodyguards. Instead of issuing sensible warnings about potential danger, they scream alarms or nag incessantly. Rather than providing security so that you are free to move through your daily life without constantly looking over your shoulder, they lock you in your room. Rather than bringing you peace of mind, they commandeer your attention until everything seems like a potential threat, making it hard to pursue what matters most to you. And once fear and anxiety take hold, it can be hard to loosen their grip.

Of course, it's only natural to respond to a warning by trying to escape the threat. Once we know that danger lurks in certain places, it's wise to steer clear. But when we listen too zealously to anxiety and fear, we can end up spending more and more time and energy fleeing and avoiding—physically, mentally, and emotionally. Our field of vision narrows; our breadth and depth of experience shrink. We become imprisoned by our self-preservation instincts, our own reactivity. To break free from anxiety's tight grip on our lives, we need to cultivate a new type of awareness—a compassionate, gentle, yet unwavering way of processing our reactions and surroundings that doesn't trigger an urge to head for the hills. This awareness is called *mindfulness*.

Mindfulness makes it possible to build a new relationship with worry and fear—to stop just surrendering to anxiety and stress. It may seem downright foolhardy to sit still when our every neuron is screaming at us to get away from whatever has set off the alarms in our body and mind—the racing heart, the tightening chest, the sense of impending doom. And yet this is the key to unlocking anxiety's hold. Our valiant efforts to *fight* anxiety, *avoid* stress, and *silence* those bossy inner body-guards are the very things preventing us from keeping our responses proportionate and useful, finding solutions for our concerns, and focus-ing our attention where it belongs: on pursuing what matters most to us in life.

The goal of this book is to help you discover how mindfulness can help you break free from your struggle with anxiety and open your life to new possibilities. We'll start by helping you build a new understand-ing of anxiety in general—where it comes from, how it operates, how it affects your life in ways you're hardly aware of. Befriending these unfa-miliar aspects of anxiety will give you a taste of mindfulness and its power to free you from a struggle that may be robbing you of life's pur-pose and meaning.

People struggle with anxiety in many ways. Some fear very spe-cific activities like public speaking or driving over bridges. Others are uncomfortable in certain situations, such as at social events or in crowded stores. You may be consumed with worry, stressed out, and tense over major life events, like the loss of a job, or minor matters, like being late for appointments. Perhaps you wrestle most with the physical symptoms—the pounding in your chest, the knot in your stomach, or overall jitteriness that sometimes come with anxiety. Or it might be the constant burden of worry and doubt that weighs you down.

Fortunately, many anxiety-related problems can be addressed through developing and applying new skills and strategies. Behavioral and cognitive-behavioral psychotherapy and self-help approaches to treating anxiety problems are, in fact, among the most successful pro-grams in the field of psychology. Yet they are not always enough. They don't help everyone, and for some people they lead to improvement but not to the comprehensive life change desired. In an attempt to address these concerns, researchers are constantly examining ways to improve these already powerful approaches.

One of the most promising of these directions, it turns out, is mindfulness. Mindfulness, with its deep roots in the Buddhist spiritual tradition, involves intentionally bringing a curious and compassionate attention to one's experiences as they are in the present moment. A recent explosion in research has been evaluating whether this kind of attention can be adapted for use in medical and mental health settings. Thanks to the pioneering work of scientists like Jon Kabat-Zinn and his colleagues at the University of Massachusetts Medical School; Marsha Linehan at the University of Washington; Steven Hayes and colleagues at the University of Nevada at Reno; Alan Marlatt at the University of Washington; and Zindel Segal, Mark Williams, and John Teasdale, we have seen that the principles and practices of mindfulness can help those struggling with chronic pain and medical conditions, depression, borderline personality disorder, addictions, and a variety of life problems. Over the last 10 years the two of us have been building on this pioneering work and looking specifically at how mindfulness can be integrated into cognitive-behavioral approaches to help those dealing with anxiety.

First we identified three common patterns of responding to anxiety that seemed to contribute to the distress and dissatisfaction associated with anxiety-related problems—that is, the patterns that seemed to turn helpful self-preservation mechanisms into metaphorical overprotective bodyguards. As you'll have a chance to see for yourself in this book, this three-part sequence involves reacting to the painful emotions of anxiety with narrowed attention and self-criticism and judgment; then trying to escape the anxiety mentally; and, finally, when that doesn't ease the discomfort, trying to avoid whatever triggers the anxiety. We have found over and over that mindfulness can reveal to someone whose attention has become chronically constricted by anxiety how these patterns unfold: how a fluttering in the chest or worrisome thought can immediately shift our attention exclusively to scanning for potential threats and how we instantly interpret this sensation, emotion, or thought as unwelcome, potentially dangerous, or a sign of inherent weakness. Mindful awareness can show us when we are trying to distract ourselves or suppress and override these thoughts, emotions, or physical sensations. It can open our eyes to how much of our life is squandered trying to skirt the people, places, and activities that could trigger anxiety.

Mindfulness practice can increase your awareness of even the most subtle cues of anxiety, allowing you to apply new skills before your emotional response escalates. Incorporating mindfulness practice into our daily lives helps us cultivate a willing stance toward anxiety, freeing us from our ongoing internal battle. Mindfulness practice helps us gain the clarity we need to take intentional actions in our life so that we are less likely to react mindlessly out of habit. It can show us how, to avoid risks, we often pass up opportunities and how we can stop focusing on avoiding anxiety more than on pursuing fulfillment.

How to Get the Most Out of This Book

Although the book is intentionally organized so that each chapter builds on the preceding one, as you probably know from your own experiences, the process of change is rarely linear. To get the most of out of this book, we recommend that you read it all the way through to build a strong foundation for change and then cycle back through the chapters to see if there are new points to be discovered or challenges to try. One of the things we find most exciting about this work is how our own understanding and connection with the material deepens each time we work with a client, supervise a therapist, apply it to our own lives, or write about it. We sincerely hope you share in that experience.

In the first three chapters of the book, we share our knowledge of fear and anxiety and how it can impair quality of life, and we provide a number of exercises designed to help you reflect on how these concepts fit your personal experience and prepare you to make the life changes you desire. The middle section of the book is aimed at helping you cultivate the foundational skills of mindfulness, build a practice that can work within the demands of your daily life, and gradually move toward bringing mindfulness to anxiety and other challenging internal states. You may want to pause a week or so between chapters in this section so that you can try out the practices and learn how they apply to your life before reading new material. The rest of the book is an invitation to engage more fully and freely with the things in life that matter most to you. In these chapters we explore how the knowledge you've gained about anxiety and the mindfulness skills you've cultivated can be used to deepen and enhance your life. We address obstacles that can cause you to veer off course and provide suggestions for how to get back on track and maintain the life changes we hope you experience. Again, taking at least a week off between chapters can give you the time you need to try out suggestions from the book and see how they relate to your own life.

The material in this book is drawn from an acceptance-based behavioral treatment program we developed for people with generalized anxiety and worry, as well as the panic, social fears, and depression that are often associated with these experiences. Given the success of the program in helping clients to both decrease their anxiety and depression and increase their quality of life, we adapted the underlying principles and exercises into this book. Through experience with our clients, we believe reading this book will lead you to reexamine how you view anxiety, other emotions, even your thoughts. This shift in perspective is extremely powerful, yet it's just a starting point for change. The way you will benefit most from what we share in this book is by applying these concepts to your life. In every chapter we have provided exercises aimed at bridging the gap between reading and living. Mindfulness is something that is experienced. It is a way of being. Our most sincere advice is to attempt all the practices we describe in the book, even if you think you know what it would be like to do them. Then, based on your own experience, you'll be able to build a practice that is right for you.

To help you build your practice, we've made audio recordings of some of the exercises we include here and posted them on a website, *www.mindfulwaythroughanxietybook.com*. It can be helpful to listen to someone lead you through specific exercises as you are learning them, so we hope these recordings will help with that process. You may also choose to record yourself reading some of them, so you can be your own guide. We also encourage you to practice at times without recordings so that you can internalize the practices and have them available to you wherever you are. This will give you flexibility and help to make mindfulness an integral part of your life.

Struggling with anxiety can be all-consuming, and it's easy to lose sight of your inner strengths and resources. Our purpose in writing this book is to help you discover the capacity you already possess to move beyond the limits that anxiety has placed on your life. Our sincere hope is that, as you read, you will develop a deeper understanding of your anxiety and related patterns of emotional response, cultivate a curious and compassionate stance toward experiences that you previously found frightening or confusing, and participate in your life in satisfying and meaningful new ways. Although the material in this book is derived from our research and clinical experience, it is also deeply personal to us. Mindfulness and the concepts we write about in this book inform how we live our personal lives, how we teach, parent, connect with friends, love our partners, and approach our own struggles. We hope you find these concepts as useful and life-enhancing as we have.

Is This Book for You?

I don't think I have an anxiety disorder or anything like that. I am just really anxious about everything going on in my life right now. Does this book make sense for me?

Although this book was informed by our research with those who have significant clinical anxiety, we believe the principles and processes described are universal. Anxiety is part of being human, and many of our first-line coping responses, like distraction or avoidance, are driven by basic biological and cultural forces. Mindfulness directly targets these common habits by increasing our awareness and allowing us to respond more flexibly.

My anxiety is pretty severe, and in the past I have been diagnosed with an anxiety disorder. Does this book make sense for me?

This book is based on and informed by the work we do with clients who struggle with significant anxiety. We think people with anxiety disorders may find it extremely relevant to their experience and helpful. If you are currently in therapy, we encourage you to talk to your therapist about mindfulness and find out how he or she thinks it may fit with the work you are already doing. If you are not in therapy, you may find that the book inspires you to seek that extra support. Finding the right therapist sometimes takes patience and perseverance. A few resources you might try are the Association for Behavioral and Cognitive Therapies (*www.abct.org*), the Anxiety Disorders Association of America (*www.adaa.org*), or the Association for Contextual Behavioral Science (*www.contextualpsychology.org*). All of these organizations have a "Find a Therapist" feature on their websites that can serve as a starting point. Feel free to try meeting with multiple therapists in order to find one whose style fits best with you. Although reading a book like this one can definitely help people with significant anxiety, we also highly recommend therapy, which can help you to personalize and apply these concepts to your own life.

Does it matter whether I am taking medication for anxiety?

A lot of people we treat are taking prescription medication for anxiety, depression, or both issues. Often they tell us that they find their emotions too intense, distressing, and life interfering and that the medication brings them some relief. Because mindfulness involves being open to, accepting, and allowing of one's experiences, however pleasant or unpleasant they may be in a given moment, it can seem like taking medication runs counter to this stance. Our opinion is that if you are contemplating medication because you are finding your anxiety uncomfortable and you want to control it, the methods described in this book may offer an alternative. If you are already on medication because you find your emotions too intense to experience, we still believe that you can use and benefit from mindfulness practice and the other concepts described in this book. Sometimes we work with clients who feel they need to be on medication for anxiety at the beginning of treatment, but as they develop a mindfulness practice they become interested in coming off the medication. If that happens to you in the course of reading the book and practicing mindfulness, we encourage you to talk with your health care provider to choose the safest and most appropriate option for you.

My anxiety comes from real-life stressors. How can this book help me?

The approach we describe can help people whose anxiety seems to come out of nowhere, as well as those whose anxiety is clearly tied to real-life stressful circumstances. Anxiety is a natural human response, and many people's lives naturally elicit a great deal of fear, stress, and anxiety. Although we would much rather be able to remove those sources of stress, we can't always do that. The approach we present can help you to respond to these real-life stressors in ways that may allow you to live your life more fully and in a more satisfying way, despite the real-life restrictions you face.

I'm trying to deal with both anxiety and depression. Will this book help me?

Depression and anxiety commonly co-occur, and many of the people we have treated have also had significant symptoms of depression. We have found that a mindful approach typically leads to a significant reduction in depressive symptoms as well. Research has shown that mindfulness can reduce depressive relapse, and effective treatments for depression often include a focus on behavioral engagement that we also present here. So our approach is very likely to help with both the depression and the anxiety you experience.

I am having other psychological problems (e.g., drinking or using substances, an eating disorder), but I also experience a great deal of anxiety. Can this book help me?

People who have difficulties with drinking, using substances, or restricting food intake often experience high levels of anxiety, either as a cause of the other difficulties, as a result of them, or both. This book may be a useful in combination with treatment or support groups that are directly aimed at the other challenges you are experiencing.

I

understanding fear and anxiety

TURNING TOWARD YOUR EMOTIONS

Marc had worked hard to create a financially secure and satisfying life. After years of college and law school, working late nights and weekends, he finally secured an enviable position at a Fortune 500 company as in-house counsel. Frequently reflecting on their early days of scrimping and saving, Marc and his wife, Janelle, truly appreciated the comfort of their beautiful suburban home, the high-quality private school education they provided for the children, and the frequent travel they enjoyed. Unfortunately, it all came crashing down on Black Thursday, the day hundreds of layoffs in the legal business were announced around the world. As the financial pressures have mounted, Marc has become increasingly nervous, irritable, and stressed. His mind is constantly busy with worry about the future and regret about the past. What if he can't find another position? Who will hire a middle-aged man in this economy? What if they lose the house? How can he explain everything to the kids? Why didn't he pursue a different career? Why didn't he save more money? All night Marc tosses and turns, his mind working through all the possible consequences of unemployment. He is exhausted from the lack of sleep and the constant tension in his neck, shoulders, and jaw.

～

It's Friday night, and the dorm is booming with activity. The hall reverberates with the competing sounds of blaring music, the whirlwind of activity in the bathroom where everyone is jockeying for a better position in front of the mirror, and the general commotion in the common area as the residents finalize their plans for the evening. Nikki turns to face the wall and pulls the covers over her head as she hears her roommate, Alisha, come back in. Alisha pauses for a moment but then, convinced that Nikki is asleep, grabs her bag and bolts out of the room to catch up with a crowd headed for the party. Nikki feels the sting of Alisha's sarcastic comment to the group—"My poor roommate seems to be coming down with the flu for the third time this month"—and she feels herself blush as peals of laughter echo through the hall. Nikki never dreamed that she would spend her weekends at college holed up alone in her room. Sure, she hadn't been a party girl in high school, but she never would have described herself as shy or anxious. Nikki had always done well in her honors classes, and she had a group of close friends who hung out together almost every weekend. But the transition to college had been rocky. Nikki was uncomfortable making new friends, and she kept to herself during orientation. Now everyone had settled into groups of friends, and she was left alone on the outside. Nikki started buying food to eat in her room because she was too embarrassed to sit alone in the cafeteria, where she imagined she would be scrutinized by all the other students. Even her schoolwork was slipping. Being organized and responsible was no longer sufficient. Nikki's professors expected her to participate regularly in class, and she had two presentations coming up. As the thoughts and images of all the possible ways she could fail as a college student flooded her mind, Nikki felt a wave of nausea overcome her. "Maybe I really am sick," she considered.

Rob carefully balanced a large cup of steaming coffee as he slid across the backseat of the pickup truck to make room for the rest of the guys on his crew. As usual, Bruce was ranting on and on about some story in the paper that had him all fired up, while George just slouched down in the seat next to him, the brim of his baseball cap pulled down low over his eyes, trying to catch a few more min-

utes of sleep before they arrived at the worksite. The conversation turned to sports, and usually Rob would have joined right in, but today he felt too jumpy to concentrate. He felt his palms start to sweat, and although he briefly thought maybe it was just the heat escaping from his cup, Rob had a sinking feeling that the constant fear he had been fighting for the last month was ramping up. Rob had been working construction for at least 20 years, and as a kid he had thought nothing of climbing up ladders or crossing beams without a safety harness. Sure, he had once seen coworkers take a bad fall, but he was confident in his own ability to stay balanced and secure. But lately Rob noticed he felt shaky and dizzy whenever he was doing roof work. He had trouble holding on to his tools because his hands were so sweaty and his heart felt like it was going to pound right out of his chest. Even though Rob was too embarrassed to refuse the coffee that Bruce brought him each day, he didn't drink it, figuring the caffeine would only make things worse. As the truck turned onto the dirt road leading up to the worksite, Rob was filled with dread. He and Mary could barely make ends meet each month without his paycheck. What would happen if his anxiety got worse and he had to quit? Who was going to hire a 45-year-old roofer who couldn't climb a ladder?

Joan is a stay-at-home mom with four children ranging in age from 6 to 15. Although all the kids are finally in school, with one in elementary, two in middle school, and a sophomore at the high school, Joan's days are easily filled. Between serving as PTO secretary, volunteering in the school library, and just keeping up with the kids' activities, Joan has little time for herself. The only appointment she always keeps is her check-in with Dr. Sedona, the psychiatrist who has been prescribing Joan medication for panic disorder for more than a decade. Joan has been anxious her whole life. As a teenager she had preferred a quiet night at home with her family to the parties and sporting events popular with her peers. At her older brother's urging Joan tried living away at college, but after only a month in the dorms she had experienced her first panic attack. Joan was reviewing her sociology textbook in preparation for a quiz when she noticed the words begin to blur and felt a wave *of dizziness and lightheadedness. When her heart began racing and she couldn't catch her breath, she asked her roommate for help and ended up at the emergency room. Six months later she was diagnosed with panic disorder. Fortunately, Joan hasn't had a panic attack in more than 10 years, but she still lives in fear that her symptoms will return, and as a result she keeps to her comfort zone. But lately Joan has begun to worry about what will happen as her kids get older and expect more of her. Her daughter is always asking to go to the mall, but Joan refuses, knowing she would feel trapped and panicky if they ventured into the middle of such a large and crowded building. And the only thing Joan's son wants for his birthday is to attend a concert. But it would be too risky to try to chaperone a group of teenagers in an unfamiliar setting she knows would set off a panic attack. Joan is worried about how she will adapt to these changes and new demands.*

If you picked up this book, you are undoubtedly struggling with something you identify as anxiety. It may be that you recently experienced an event that has left you incredibly anxious, like the loss of a job. Or maybe you're going through a big life transition such as divorce or graduation from college. Perhaps you just noticed that anxiety has been gradually creeping into different aspects of your life, making it harder for you to live the way you want, leaving you exhausted, stressed, and overwhelmed. Maybe you've battled anxiety your entire life and wonder if significant change is possible. Or maybe you've always experienced a lot of stress and worry but viewed it as integral to your success in life, and only lately have you begun to wonder whether there is another way of being in the world.

Whatever your circumstances, through your personal experiences you likely know a lot about this emotional state—how it feels, what situations are likely to bring it on, and, perhaps most painfully, the toll it can take on your life.

We too have some expertise in understanding fear and anxiety, from our own personal experiences, but also from our extensive research and clinical work in this area. That's why we hope you'll allow yourself to learn from our mistakes as you read this chapter and the rest of the book. The faces of anxiety we just showed you may not fully capture what you're going through. Later in the book we might recommend particular coping strategies that seem counterintuitive or that don't immediately strike you as likely to be effective for you. We know (somewhat painfully) from our own experience that sometimes all of us prematurely judge and dismiss information that doesn't fit with how we typically view ourselves and the world. Even as psychologists who study and practice mindfulness—a special type of awareness that allows us to observe our internal states as well as our environment with gentle curiosity and compassion, through a clear, wide-angle lens—we are constantly amazed by the things we learn about our own reactions and behaviors when we allow ourselves to fully consider new and foreign ideas and options.

So, as we present the scientifically and clinically derived general knowledge about fear and anxiety in this chapter, we ask that you carefully consider each point to determine how it fits with your experience. We've discovered that turning toward your internal emotional experiences and making connections between what is known in the field of psychology about fear and anxiety and your own private struggles is an important step toward easing your suffering and living life more freely and fully. Every reader is unique, and we firmly believe that you're the best expert on what is right for you. Give yourself a chance to identify it.

Although the evidence suggests that bringing this new and deepened awareness called *mindfulness* to fear and anxiety ultimately reduces distress and provides new opportunities, it may seem like a strange thing to do when you're trying to reduce your anxiety. You're already painfully familiar with your emotions—wouldn't learning to ignore them be much more useful? Anxiety can be extremely uncomfortable, so it's natural to want to turn away from rather than toward it. But as we've said, even people who know a lot about anxiety (including those who study and write books on the topic) are sometimes confused by their reactions or unaware of some of the subtleties. An enhanced understanding and awareness of anxiety alleviates a lot of distress and confusion and can often make anxiety itself less overwhelming. So, even though it may require a leap of faith, we recommend that you give the exercises described in this chapter a try. At first you may find that focusing on anxiety and fear makes you feel somewhat more uncomfortable or nervous. That is a natural and normal part of the process. As you incorporate the strategies we present throughout the book, we hope you'll see a decrease in your discomfort and distress with these emotions.

EXERCISE **What do you know about fear and anxiety?**

Take a few minutes to consider your thoughts and reactions to the following questions. If you are willing, we recommend jotting down your responses in a notebook.

1. What is your anxiety like? How do you know when you're anxious?

2. What is the difference between fear and anxiety?

3. Are these emotions adaptive? If so, why do so many people struggle with anxiety?

4. What is an anxiety disorder? How does someone develop a disorder?

How Do We Know When We Are Anxious?

Claire just moved from Oklahoma to Los Angeles to take a job with an advertising firm. The weekend before she was scheduled to start, her boss invited the advertising group to dinner. Claire sat silent and wooden in her chair, surrounded by a group of young, stylish men and women engaged in animated conversation. Her ears rang with the clatter of silverware and plates and the buzz of conversation punctuated by shrieks and peals of laughter. She watched the waiters deftly move among the crowded tables of the trendy restaurant, delivering eclectic dishes to the eager diners. The minutes ticked past as Claire frantically searched for something to add to the conversation. She felt her anxiety escalating. Thoughts such as "They must think I am a total hick," "I am sure they regret hiring me," "I have to stop sitting here like an idiot and say something," and "I will never fit in here" raced through her mind. She felt a blush creep up her neck, reddening her pale skin, beads of sweat moistened her palms, and her mouth was as dry as cotton. In addition to feeling afraid and embarrassed, she felt a wave of sadness as memories of her friends and family back home passed through her mind. Abruptly Claire stood up and weaved through the crowd toward the bathroom. Moments later her boss came through the door and asked in a kind and concerned voice if Claire was ill. From the privacy of the stall, Claire steadied her voice and through her tears responded, "I think something I ate made me ill. Please apologize to everyone, but I think I better slip out of here and head home."

EXERCISE **What are your personal signs and symptoms of anxiety?—Part A**

You probably remember different times when you were anxious or situations that made you stressed at the time. For this exercise, we ask that you reflect on an anxious situation in what might be a slightly different way. Think about a time within the last week when you were fearful or anxious. After you finish reading all of these instructions, close your eyes and replay the situation in your mind as vividly as you can, almost like you are starring in your own movie. Picture the environment you were in, including any sights and sounds around you, except this time, rather than just experiencing the event as it unfolds, see if you can carefully observe your reactions, even if they are totally familiar to you. Bring a new curiosity to your examination. As you put yourself back into the situation, see if you can notice the thoughts that ran through your mind, any physical changes you noticed in your body, and any other emotions besides fear and anxiety that you experienced. Notice your behaviors—things you said or did in the situation. Try to stay with the image for several minutes, then jot down what you notice by making a list of your different responses in each domain (i.e., thoughts, physical changes, emotions, and behaviors). You may want to use a notebook to do this and the other exercises in the book so that you can keep all your responses together.

As Claire's story demonstrates, signs and symptoms of fear and anxiety appear across all our response systems. Images or memories pop into our mind, thoughts are generated, physical changes occur, emotions arise, and behavioral habits kick in. The specific response we have to an anxiety-eliciting situation is determined by many factors. Elements of the situation, our basic biology or temperament, and our personal history and learning influence our reactions. Different people approach a feared situation in different ways. For example, imagine a person receives an e-mail Sunday night to report to the boss's office first thing in the morning; a customer has filed a serious complaint. Someone who grew up with a chronically ill parent may cope with his anxious apprehension about the meeting by calling in sick to work. Another person might preemptively quit to avoid harsh criticism. Still another might "white knuckle" her way through the meeting, steeling herself against each wave of anxiety. Becoming aware of **your** unique signs and symptoms and the situations that elicit them is an important first step toward change.

Although fear and anxiety are expressed through several channels of responding—cognitive, emotional, imaginal, physical, and behavioral—we don't always notice the varied aspects of our responses. Usually we define our anxiety using a few key symptoms. For example, someone might be very aware that his mouth becomes dry every time he is called on in class. Someone else is tuned in to the way her heart races whenever she approaches or drives over a bridge. If our attention becomes focused narrowly on one or two typical or dominant responses, it is easy to miss more subtle reactions. When we are able to identify our more subtle reactions, we can catch our anxiety earlier and choose how to respond to it more effectively. For many people, physical symptoms are the easiest to notice. Stepping back and observing our thoughts when we feel anxious can be more difficult. Most of us are not used to treating thoughts as responses; we simply experience them as part of our identity. Observing emotions can also be challenging. Fear and anxiety easily grab our attention and tend to overshadow other emotions like sadness or shame that may also be present and important to notice. Behavioral responses can be both obvious and subtle. Someone might know that she avoids public speaking to keep her anxiety at bay but be less aware that she drinks three glasses of wine each night to avoid lying awake in bed, caught in a web of worry. A salesman who drives the back roads instead of the freeway to avoid the panicky feeling that comes up when tankers thunder by might convince himself that taking the alter-

> *We're usually aware of only a few key symptoms of our anxiety.*

nate route is a simple matter of preference. Noticing our subtle signs of avoidance is an important step toward reclaiming our lives.

Another characteristic of anxiety that is not always apparent is how responses in one domain can trigger responses in another. While reviewing notes an hour before a test, a student might have the thought, "I am not prepared for this exam." This thought can set off a chain reaction of physical symptoms like tightness in his chest and rapid, shallow breathing. Increasing his rate of breathing naturally causes his heart to pump faster, which signals to him that he is really getting anxious now. Noticing these physical sensations prompts a cascade of thoughts about how scary and uncomfortable it is to be anxious and how anxiety will surely interfere with his performance on the test. These thoughts prompt the student to close his book abruptly and leave the library in an attempt to escape any cue that might increase the intensity of his fear. In this way, our anxious responses feed one another in an increasing spiral. Often we do not notice the signs until they are already quite intense and overwhelming, making it much harder to respond effectively to our anxiety.

> *Our anxious responses feed each other so quickly that by the time we notice the anxiety it feels out of control.*

How can we both be aware that we are struggling with anxiety and also miss some of its signs? Moving toward and paying close attention to painful experiences is not something we are naturally inclined to do. Have you ever done something really embarrassing? We certainly have! And when a memory of what we said or did comes up, often we want to scream "NO!" and push that image right out of our mind. It can be really uncomfortable to remember how we put our foot in our mouth, to relive turning red, to recall the look on the other person's face. Part of being human is that we are driven to avoid painful experiences. Although this natural tendency toward avoidance is protective, it makes it difficult to notice subtleties in the cascade of responses that make up anxiety. Also, anxious responses often occur quickly and automatically, like an ingrained habit, outside of our focus of awareness.

At the other end of the spectrum, sometimes we dwell on anxious events. We might replay a situation over and over in our mind. Our clients are often surprised, and a bit skeptical, when we suggest that the first step to living a fuller life involves carefully observing anxiety each time is arises. Many people who struggle with anxiety already feel that they are painfully aware of their signs and symptoms.

Purposefully observing our reaction to an anxiety-provoking situation is qualitatively different from our typical way of noticing. If our initial reaction to an anxious thought or a frightening image is to wince and turn away, purposefully observing involves bringing our attention back to it. If our initial reaction is "been there, done that," like listening to a broken record—same thing over and over again—the challenge is to look closer and see if we can find some part of our anxious response that we hadn't noticed before.

> *Mindful awareness of the full experience of anxiety can help us see it coming and manage it better.*

This method of observation—**turning toward something that we would usually avoid** and **taking a fresh look at a familiar response**—is a key characteristic of mindfulness, a core skill we hope to help you develop as you work through this book. Mindfulness involves other skills as well, but cultivating a new way of observing is the first step.

EXERCISE **What are your personal signs and symptoms of anxiety?—Part B**

Consider the list below and find the signs and symptoms that you typically experience with anxiety. You may also want to note those that you haven't necessarily noticed but you think may be worth looking for as we move forward. It may be helpful to jot these down in your notebook so that you can remember to notice them as they occur during the day.

Thoughts

Worries about what might occur in the future (*e.g.*, *"I will fail this test," "I will be uncomfortable at the party," "My children will not be happy," "My parents will become ill," "I will have a panic attack in the supermarket," "I am going to get sick from the germs in this bathroom"*)

Ruminations about the past (*e.g.*, *"I can't believe I said that," "My boss was so disappointed in me," "I wish I hadn't snapped at my partner that way," "Running into that dog in the park was terrifying"*)

Thoughts about being in danger (*e.g.*, *"I can't do this," "I am having a heart attack," "I am losing my mind"*)

Critical thoughts about the self (*e.g., "I am such an idiot," "I am so lazy," "I'm such a procrastinator," "I am a total loser," "I am a failure"*)

Other thoughts?

Physical sensations

Rapid heart rate

Dizziness or lightheadedness

Sweating

Shortness of breath

Blushing

Trembling or shaky feelings

Dry mouth

Stomach distress

Tension or soreness in the neck, shoulders, or any other muscles

Headaches

Restlessness

Fatigue

Irritability

Other sensations?

Additional emotions

Anger

Sadness

Surprise

Disgust

Shame

Other emotions?

Behaviors

Repetitive behaviors or habits (*e.g., biting fingernails, tapping feet, playing with hair*)

Avoidance or escape (*e.g., turning down an invitation; passing up a promotion; calling in sick to work; making an excuse to cancel a social engagement; leaving an event early; asking someone else to make a phone call for you; taking an alternative route to avoid a bridge, tunnel, or other landmark; using a ritual, security object, or lucky charm to get through an anxious experience)*

Distraction techniques *(e.g., overeating, smoking, watching television, having a few glasses of wine or a couple of beers, sleeping, shopping)*

Attempts to gain power or protect oneself *(e.g., communicate aggression, threaten others, assert dominance, express anger)*

Other behaviors?

How Does Anxiety Differ from Fear?

Imagine driving through the countryside on a warm, sunny fall afternoon. The trees are ablaze with red and yellow leaves, accented by a brilliant blue sky. A calm peacefulness envelops you as you travel the gently sloping road. Suddenly an eighteen-wheeler comes into view, careening toward you on the wrong side of the road. Your heart jumps into your throat, and you swerve onto the shoulder just in time for the truck to go roaring by, shaking your car with its force. You break out into a sweat, your heart races, and you feel like someone just punched you in the gut.

Fear is a natural and helpful alarm that alerts us to potentially dangerous situations. When we detect a threat, our nervous system immediately kicks into gear and sets off a cascade of responses all aimed to ready us for action. The parts of our brains that respond to threat react automatically, without involving the parts of our brains involved in deliberation or more complex thought. The rate and strength of our heartbeat increases to move oxygen to large muscles in our arms and legs more efficiently and effectively to help us respond effectively to an emergency. At the same time, the current of our blood flow moves away from places where it is less needed (the brain, fingers, and toes) and toward our large muscles. The pupils in our eyes dilate so that we can scan our environment for threats. All of these changes, known as the *fight-or-flight response*, are aimed at preparing us to either fight off a threat or flee to safety. The physical symptoms of fear that we experience when these changes occur (rapid heartbeat, increased breathing, dizziness) are simply the side effects of our body readying itself for action. Fear can also elicit what is known as the *freeze response*. This happens when we don't respond at all in a dangerous situation in the hope that the threat will pass. For example in the wild, if a rabbit senses a predator, such as a fox, it becomes immobile to minimize the chances of detection and capture. Humans can also experience the freeze response under conditions of extreme fear. Consider how we sometimes describe feeling "petrified" or like a statue. For example, an accident victim may remain seated in her car even when freed from the rubble and directed toward safety.

Physical threats are not the only danger cues humans are built to avoid. Sensitivity to possible social threats in our environment is another hardwired survival response. Both animals and humans depend on a larger community for safety and security. For example, wolves survive by earning their place in the structure and hierarchy of a pack. A heightened awareness of social cues is essential for successful integration and acceptance into a group or society.

Because fear of physical and social threats is critical to our survival, this response system is remarkably well developed. It works quickly and effectively without requiring any thought or purposeful effort on our part. Having such an efficient fear response is extremely beneficial. We have a much better chance of survival if we are instantly prepared to defend ourselves against outside threat.

Now imagine that at the end of the week you are responsible for a big presentation at work. Your unit has been underperforming and there is rumor of layoffs. The CEO and VP from corporate are flying out to hear your explanation. Unfortunately, you were alerted to this visit only 3 days ago, and you don't feel like you have had adequate time to prepare. Worse, every time you get a few hours to work on the presentation your mind either goes blank or spins off in a million directions. You just cannot concentrate. Your shoulders, neck, and jaw are tight with tension, and there is nothing you can do to loosen those muscles. At home, you feel cranky and irritable. You race through the kids' bedtime story because your mind is filled with budget projections and workload distribution. When you think about the actual presentation, you imagine stumbling over your words, not being able to answer important questions, and letting your whole unit down. You think about all the people whose jobs depend on your ability to get this right.

Compared to fear, anxiety is a more subtle but chronic state. Whereas fear is an automatic response to a threat we perceive as imminent, anxiety involves thinking about or imagining some threat that we could encounter in the future. With fear our response is automatic; there is little need for higher-level thinking. We don't ponder whether to step out of oncoming traffic; we simply react. In contrast, anxiety is defined primarily by anticipation.

When we are faced with a threat, we feel a surge of fear that peaks in a matter of moments and begins to subside when we are safe. In contrast, an anxious response lingers as we consider and prepare for future possibilities. As a result, anxiety is associated with a general sense of restlessness and irritability. Remaining continuously poised for a possible threat can produce muscle tension, especially in the shoulders, neck, and face. Because our minds are busy considering the future, it is difficult to concentrate on the present while anxious. These cognitive and physical symptoms often disrupt our sleep, leaving us feeling worn out or exhausted.

> *Anxiety is defined mainly by anticipation.*

Although prolonged anxiety can take a significant toll on our physical and mental well-being, the ability to consider possible future threats and prepare for them can also boost self-preservation and success. Considering what sort of questions might be on a test is a useful way to prepare. Imagining a physical challenge that lies ahead can prompt us to exercise and train. Envisioning the damage a hurricane might cause can help us make the necessary arrangements to stay safe.

	Fear versus	**Anxiety**
Nature of threat	Immediate	Future
Physical response	Surge of panic	Chronic tension and arousal
Function	Survival	Preparedness

Are These Emotions Helpful?

We are hardwired for fear because it helps us respond to physical and social threats and increases the chances of our survival. We share this basic instinct for survival with many other species. But as humans, we also have some unique characteristics that sometimes disrupt this primitive survival response and cause us stress. The very same attributes that allow us to imagine, problem-solve, plan, and reminisce make it possible for us to be consumed with relentless anxiety.

We can think, remember, and vividly imagine innumerable threats.

Humans do not need to be confronted with a real, immediate physical or social threat to feel fear. Totally absorbed in a good book or engaging movie, we feel suspense and apprehension mount as the lead character enters the darkened room and full-blown fear when the villain attacks, even though we know we are safe. The human mind is sort of like a cinema that never closes. Awake or asleep, we can vividly imagine all sorts of potential threats and feared outcomes. We can also rerun an infinite number of past occasions marked by fear and anxiety. Our minds are excellent at conjuring up extremely realistic portrayals of these events.

> *The human mind is like a movie theater that never closes—always prepared to show films of what we fear.*

To make matters worse, we don't usually rehash embarrassing incidents or imagine future disasters with detachment and objectivity. Just imagining or remembering an event can bring up a flood of anxious thoughts and physical sensations and encourage behaviors such as distraction or escape. Anxiously awaiting her son's return 2 hours past curfew and imagining a fatal car crash, a mother can suffer the same stomach distress, sweaty palms, and dry mouth she would at the scene of the accident. Lying in bed recalling a botched class presentation, the high school student can experience the same heart palpitations that he endured during class.

The ability to remember and imagine is an extremely valuable human characteristic that has allowed our society to advance in significant ways. Unfortunately, it also grants us unlimited access to an infinite number of feared events. Encountering an endless stream of threats in our minds significantly complicates the fear response, which on its own functions as a basic biological survival system.

Our ability to vividly imagine threats also tricks our brains into

> *Mindfulness can help us know when we're experiencing fear and when it's anxiety— and how to respond.*

thinking that these threats are more likely to occur. Research has shown that people estimate that events are more likely to happen when they can easily visualize them. Evolutionarily, this tendency was protective because, before the advent of photographs, people could more readily picture events they had recently seen in their own environment, meaning these events were, in fact, more likely. If a villager could recall a vivid image of someone getting sick from eating berries, avoiding similar-looking berries was a good idea. But in the modern age of 24-hour news coverage and cell phone video recordings of every tragic event around the globe, we can readily imagine tsunamis, earthquakes, flu epidemics, child abductions, and terrorist attacks, no matter how unlikely they are in our surroundings. Our once-adaptive tendency leaves us vulnerable to a cascade of media-induced fears.

We know there is a future, and we want to control it.

One uncomfortable truth about being human is that we know there is a future and it is uncertain. If we knew exactly what was in store for us, our ability to think ahead and plan could prevent us from falling victim to all sorts of dangers. If we knew a disgruntled coworker would go on a shooting rampage on a particular day, we could stay home, warn our friends, and call the police. If we could predict the future with crystal-clear accuracy, developing a detailed defensive strategy would be well worth the investment of time and mental effort. But given the uncertainty and uncontrollability of the future, such planning is impossible. Effort might be wasted planning for an event that never actually occurred. Or a seemingly well-thought-out plan could go awry because of circumstances beyond our control.

> *Jade spent hours preparing for a big exam. She faithfully attended class, kept up with the reading, and participated in the study group. Jade created a comprehensive study guide and carefully reviewed it the weekend before the test. In other words, she imagined what taking a final exam would be like and tried her best to prepare for it. Unfortunately, imagining and preparing for an event is not the same as controlling it. What if Jade's teacher is unreasonable and creates an unfair exam? What if Jade is involved in an accident on the way to school the morning of her exam? What if she develops a*

migraine during the test? What if her concentration is disturbed by a classmate's sniffling and sneezing?

Planning and preparing for events in the future is a wise and adaptive strategy. But, as is often paraphrased from the poet Robert Burns, "The best laid schemes of mice and men, go often askew." Part of being human is managing the balance between anticipating the future and accepting its uncertainty. Worry is a sign that the balance has been disrupted.

> *Worry is a sign of imbalance between anticipating the future and accepting its uncertainty.*

Worry versus problem solving—how do you tell them apart?

Worry differs from problem solving in a few subtle but important ways. Often we worry about problems that haven't actually happened yet, which makes it difficult to come up with and implement a viable solution. Also, we tend to worry about things we can't actually control, which means that no matter how hard we search, or how creative we are, there is no solution that we can enact. Sometimes we worry and ruminate about problems when we are unwilling to take the actions that would be necessary to solve the problem. Worry can sometimes be how we express love and concern, like when a family member is struggling with a chronic illness. But despite our intentions, being consumed with worry can sometimes strain our relationships by preventing us from fully connecting with the people we care about. Although the processes of problem solving and worry look deceptively similar on the surface, problem solving moves us closer to a resolution, whereas worry keeps us spinning in an endless cycle.

Another unique characteristic of worry is that sometimes it is the process, rather than the actual content, that is important to pay attention to. Sometimes we develop a worry habit, such that we approach all kinds of problems with the same anxious apprehension. One sign that we are deeply entrenched in the worry habit is when the focus of the problem to be solved or the threat to be avoided constantly shifts. So one might start the day worrying about running late for work, then refocus on worry over a report that is due, and on the way home worry about getting through a list of chores. In the moment we might be consumed with one worry (running late), but as soon as the problem is resolved a new worry pops up to take its place. Humans can imagine an endless list of problems, which require the continuous generation of solutions. If we are not willing to accept that some elements of the future are beyond our control, some problems unsolvable, we can get pulled into an endless cycle of preparing for any and all possibilities—as Maria was when she heard a news report predicting an overnight blizzard.

Maria searched the Internet for updates on the weather as she anxiously awaited a call from her husband, Bob. She had texted him earlier with news of the storm, hoping he would help her develop a plan for the morning. After about 15 minutes the phone rang, bringing good news. Bob had made arrangements with the couple's next-door neighbor Doris, who was available to watch their daughter, Kate, if school was canceled. Maria felt a wave of relief, but as she prepared dinner she began to worry about whether she was too reliant on Doris for help: "What if she resents our asking? In the last month I have asked her to watch Kate twice, and we borrowed her snow blower. What if she thinks we're a bunch of freeloaders?" Maria picked up the phone and called Bob for reassurance. "Doris was fine with watching Kate," Bob assured his wife. "I think she is looking forward to the company. She said they could drink hot cocoa, play games, and even make a batch of chocolate chip cookies together." At first the conversation soothed Maria's fears, but as she reflected on Bob's words, a slew of new worries emerged. "What kind of parent am I? I can't remember the last time I sat down with Kate to play a game. And we haven't baked together since she was in kindergarten. Maybe I should take the day off from work. But what if my boss gets upset? I just took a vacation day last week. And Doris might be offended if I cancel. What if she thinks I don't trust her? But after all, she is getting older. Does she have the energy to care for Kate? What if she falls asleep while they're watching television and Kate is unsupervised? What if Kate tries to get the cookies out of the oven and burns herself?" Maria's thoughts were interrupted by the thump of a car door. She glanced up and was startled to see that it was 6:30, Bob and Kate were home, and she hadn't even started dinner.

In contrast, Maria's friend Cassie acknowledges that an overnight snowstorm could close her daughter's school and complicate her commute to work. To prepare (or problem-solve), she arranges for alternative child care and sets her alarm to go off an hour early to allow for extra time in the morning. By addressing a finite number of problems, Cassie avoids getting pulled into the vortex of anxiety.

Worrying is not a pleasant experience. It consumes our time, interferes with our concentration, and generally leaves us tense and exhausted. Worry pulls us into the future and distracts us from what is happening in the present. If during breakfast we mentally review all the problems we may need to tackle at work, we'll find it hard to savor the meal or appreciate the company of our family. If talking with someone we are attracted to sets our mind racing to fears of possible rejection, we won't be able to establish a connection with that person in the moment. If we worry incessantly about the well-being and security of our family, and thus are too keyed up and on edge to enjoy our time with them, we may inadvertently undermine the very relationships we are working so hard to preserve.

We also struggle with worry because it seems to occur outside our control. It seems as if fears of "what if?" take our attention hostage and prevent us from focusing on what matters to us personally. Surprisingly, research suggests that worry can serve a purpose, even if we usually don't do it intentionally. At first, this idea may seem ridiculous and even invalidating. It may sound as though we can just choose to stop worrying if we are doing it for a reason. If you've struggled at all with worry, your experience probably tells you that it's not that simple. But understanding that worry is a habit supported and strengthened by rewards is an important first step toward loosening its grip on your life.

Every action we engage in as humans has a function or purpose. Even behaviors that we know could harm us in some way, like smoking cigarettes or eating junk food, provide some reward in that they typically serve some positive function. For example, smoking is associated with an increased risk for cancer, but it also serves as a stress reliever. Eating junk food is unhealthy and associated with long-term weight gain, yet it can also provide a temporary refuge from stress or just the momentary pleasure of eating something that tastes good. Unfortunately, reaping the rewards of such a behavior reinforces it, making us more likely to continue doing it. And so the vicious cycle begins. the rewards influence our actions outside of our intentions, making these habits particularly hard to break.

EXERCISE **What is the function of worry?**

Often we are so distracted by and caught up in our worries that we don't even stop to consider the purpose of our worry. As you become more aware and mindful of your worry and anxiety, these functions may become clearer. But for now we would like you just to reflect on some possible reasons that you worry. As you read over the list below, consider which items might represent the function or functions of worry for you.

- To prepare for some imagined future event
- To make sure I think through all my options and pick the right or perfect solution to a problem
- To figure out whether there is any solution besides the one that requires me to do or say something I am uncomfortable about
- To feel like I am doing something about a problem even though I may not actually have control over it
- To stop something bad from happening, even though I know it is out of my control
  — Superstition: "If I worry, it is less likely to happen."
  — Protection: "If I think things through enough, I can prevent something from happening."
- To motivate myself to do something I don't feel like doing
- To avoid thinking about and feeling bad about something else

Many of the reasons we feel compelled to worry can be categorized as attempts to gain control over or brace ourselves for some aspect of the future. For example, Gina worries about her boyfriend leaving her so that she won't be sad and lonely if he does. Erin worries about her auditions to prevent herself from feeling disappointed if she doesn't land a role. Unfortunately, it is painful when someone we love leaves us, or when we are disappointed or let down in some way. Worrying can seem like a way to brace ourselves against possible pain, but as we will discuss later, this approach often backfires.

Worrying to stop something bad from happening is a behavior that is reinforced and strengthened over time. If Margaret worries about her daughter Alyson, hoping the worry will protect Alyson from contracting swine flu, and Alyson remains healthy, Margaret will learn that her worrying protects her family. In other words, Alyson's clean bill of health rewards Margaret for worrying. Worries about events that are extremely improbable (your plane crashing, your fainting in public, or developing a terminal disease) are often maintained this way.

Sometimes it seems like worrying about a negative outcome will motivate us to prepare for it. For example, Jake worries about failing every exam because he thinks the anxiety and fear his worry produces will encourage him to study. Some anxious apprehension can be helpful in focusing our attention and increasing our adrenaline. But, ironically, the anxious responses characteristic of someone who struggles with pervasive and severe worry usually act as obstacles to adequate preparation. If studying is associated with images of failure, harsh and critical self-judgments, shame, and guilt, Jake will be motivated to avoid it.

You might be wondering why Jake doesn't realize that worry is not working as a motivator. It may be that Jake knows worrying is not motivating him to study, but he blames himself for his failures rather than considering that the strategy may be ineffective. Human behavior is influenced more strongly by the rules we have about how things are supposed to work than by our actual experience. If Jake has learned directly or indirectly that imagining the consequences of failure is the best way to ensure success, he most likely will continue to worry despite new evidence to the contrary.

> *Why do we keep worrying that extremely rare events will occur when we see repeatedly that they don't? Because we think it was our worrying that staved them off.*

Investigating why people worry has become a focus of interest among psychological researchers. One line of research is aimed at examining whether occasional and problem worriers differ in the reasons they give for worrying. Worrying to avoid negative outcomes and prepare for the future is common across all worriers. Only one reason for worrying was found to be more common among problem worriers. That group reported that they sometimes worried about "minor" matters to avoid thinking about and feeling emotions related to other, more distressing life concerns. For example, Tom worries about the condition of his lawn and keeping his shed organized and his gutters meticulously clean to avoid facing some significant problem in his marriage. Similarly, Marissa worries about being late to appointments, asking for directions, and returning items to a store, but she avoids thinking about how lonely she has been since she moved into her own apartment.

> *One difference between problem worriers and occasional worriers: Problem worriers worry about minor matters to avoid dwelling on more distressing matters.*

To summarize, fear is an extremely useful emotion that maximizes our chances of survival. But our uniquely human ability to imagine future threats, and our natural desire to want to control or avoid them, puts us at risk for chronic worry and anxiety. Worry is often rewarded or reinforced, so once the habit is established it can be difficult to break.

Fear **prepares** us to respond in self-protective ways but does not **require** us to do so.

Sometimes our desire to pursue what is personally meaningful may conflict with our biological programming. When we sense a threat, our alarm system readies us for action. We are alerted to possible threat, and we experience physical changes that prepare us to run, fight, or freeze. But a number of personal and environmental factors will influence how we ultimately respond to this potential threat. One significant factor is our personal values or what we find meaningful and fulfilling.

Let's say you feel a surge of fear as you wait for a job interview. This fear is delivering a message: what you are about to do is important ... be alert ... there is some risk here. A number of behavioral responses to this alarm are possible. You can leave. You can try to distract yourself from your feelings, or talk yourself out of being anxious. Or you can acknowledge the message and choose to go ahead with the interview because what's meaningful to you in this

> *Mindful awareness can help us see when we want to override our biological programming and ignore the warnings issued by fear and anxiety. Always heeding these warnings without question can lead to chronic anxiety and restrict our lives.*

situation is the recognition that you can't get a better-paying or more rewarding job without taking risks. And you can't take risks without feeling some anxiety or fear.

Likewise, the first time you share your true feelings with an intimate partner, it is completely natural to feel afraid. This emotion alerts you that you are vulnerable in this situation—you could be rejected. Yet you may choose to take the risk because being close to others is something you value.

We are constantly challenged to take risks in life domains that we value, such as relationships and work. Our biological programming ensures that these risks will elicit anxious reactions—feelings of vulnerability, anxiety, insecurity, uncertainty about the future. This alarm reaction sets off a series of physical changes that focus our attention and prepare us to defend ourselves or to escape danger. However, in the pursuit of a meaningful and fulfilling life we may choose to override these behavioral tendencies.

What Is an Anxiety Disorder?

If feeling fear and anxiety is a normal part of being human, how much anxiety is too much? When does "normal" worrying become an anxiety disorder?

- Does worrying every day signal the presence of a disorder?
- Is it normal to blush every time you enter a social situation?
- If you were told in the emergency room that you had a panic attack, does that mean you have a chronic psychological condition?
- Is checking to see if the doors are locked at night even though you know you already locked them normal?
- If anxiety and worry run in your family, are you destined to live with an anxiety disorder as a chronic condition because it's in your genes?

Although fear and anxiety are normal human responses, psychology and psychiatry have come to recognize certain specific anxiety disorders (a quick overview of each disorder appears below). Each anxiety disorder is marked by a unique set of signs and symptoms, but these disorders are not defined solely by the amount or type of anxiety felt. We all differ in our basic temperaments, and some of us are more inclined to respond to situations with apprehension or fear. Someone can be a self-defined worrier, blush in almost every social situation, be prone to occasional panic attacks, or frequently think irrational, anxious thoughts without meeting the criteria for an anxiety disorder. There is one important feature that all anxiety disorders share: the presence of significant **distress** and/or *life interference*. When you become seriously troubled by your anxious reactions and/or they prevent you from engaging in important life activities, you may be struggling with an anxiety disorder.

> *Dina has out-of-the-blue panic attacks, which involve a surge of intense fear, several times a year. Although the attacks are uncomfortable and inconvenient, she is not particularly bothered or alarmed by their occurrence. She hasn't made any changes to her work or recreational habits, and the panic attacks don't have any impact on her relationships. In contrast, Christina had one panic attack approximately 8 months ago. It was a horrible experience for her, and she is terrified that it will happen again. In fact, Christina is no longer willing to shop in the supermarket alone. She either waits for her partner to accompany her or picks up what she needs at the local convenience store. Although both women experience panic attacks, only Christina would meet the criteria for an anxiety disorder.*
>
> *Similarly, Sarah feels nervous when she has to do a scientific presentation. At the beginning her mouth is usually dry and her voice a bit shaky. Sometimes she has thoughts such as "I don't have anything important to say" and "The audience can tell I am anxious." But Sarah accepts that these responses are a pretty normal part of public speaking, especially for someone who is a bit shy. Despite the presence of anxious thoughts that say otherwise, Sarah believes she has something important to contribute to her field and values sharing the results of her work with other scientists. Sarah regularly accepts invitations to present her work at conferences around the country. On the other hand, Ivan wishes he could present his work, but he feels like his anxiety gets in the way. The few times he has agreed to speak at a conference, he noticed signs of*

*anxiety creeping up as soon as he pulled his materials together. Each time, he apologized to the conference organizer, claiming he was too ill to present. Ivan's view is that he can be an effective speaker only if he is anxiety-free. Because of this, he has passed up several opportunities to participate in scientific conferences, and he is concerned about his chances of getting tenure. Both Sarah and Ivan experience some fear of public speaking, but Ivan's **response** to his fear, characterized by distress and avoidance, suggests that he may have an anxiety disorder.*

Whether you have been diagnosed with an anxiety disorder, you notice symptoms across disorders that seem relevant to you, or you are just concerned about the role of anxiety and fear in your life given the stressors you face, our goal is to help you change the relationship you have with these emotions. Mindfulness practice can reduce the pain and suffering many of us experience in response to fear and anxiety and provide us some freedom to pursue the life directions that matter most. Becoming aware of the nature and function of fear, anxiety, and worry is the first step toward living a mindful and engaged life.

EXERCISE **Turning toward your emotions: Paying attention to fear and anxiety in a new way**

Over the next few days we would like you to observe your response when you notice yourself beginning to feel anxious or afraid. This method of observation involves *turning toward something that we would usually avoid and taking a fresh look at a familiar response.* Most likely you have developed a strong habit of reacting to your anxiety with negative judgment and self-criticism, and you probably put a lot of effort into ignoring it or pushing it away. The goal of this book is to promote a radically different way of responding to painful emotions. Naturally, establishing a new habit takes time and practice. At the end of each chapter, after you have been introduced to a new concept related to mindfulness, we suggest an observational practice for you to try. These practices are designed to be progressively more challenging and complex, yet every step is important. A very subtle but critical first step to changing your relationship with anxiety is to prac tice simply noticing anxious responses when they arise and observing them just as they are. Although it can seem uncomfortable and perhaps unnecessary, we highly recommend that you carry a small notebook and record your responses in it. At this point, just noting the day, the situation you are in, and any anxious responses you notice would be an extremely helpful first step. So you might notice physical sensations, thoughts, or behaviors—just note whatever you are aware of in the moment you realize you are anxious. Below is a list of *common questions* that people often have when they think about recording their experiences in this way.

Do I have to write things down while I'm in the situation? That seems difficult or embarrassing. Can't I wait until later?

We strongly recommend noting your responses while you are still feeling anxious. In fact, the earlier you notice anxiety and take a moment to record it, the better. One of the goals of this exercise is to break into the automatic, habitual cycle of anxiety. We want you to develop a new habit, which involves taking a mental step back *while* you are anxious to check in with your experience.

Do I need to mark something down every time I'm anxious? I'd be writing all day.

We want you to develop some experience with noticing your anxiety in a new way. And the more frequently you record your reactions, the sooner you will break your old habits and begin building new ones. You can decide the pace you want to take (we certainly understand how life can get very busy). We recommend that you stop and record your experience at least once a day as you are reading through the book, although you will benefit more from doing so more frequently. As your new habit develops, try alternating between physically recording your reactions in the notebook and mentally completing the steps.

What if I can't observe thoughts or behaviors?

Observing your experience takes a lot of practice. We teach you new ways to develop this skill throughout the book. In the meantime, read over the exercise "*What are your personal signs and symptoms of anxiety?—Part B*" (pages 18–20) and see if you notice any of the responses described there.

Won't purposely paying attention to my anxiety make me more anxious?

Since you bought this book, we assume you're already paying some attention to your anxiety. Still, you may feel somewhat more anxious as you initially turn toward your anxiety by noticing and recording it. If you're used to ignoring your emotions, you may feel uncomfortable noticing how often anxiety appears. It's important to understand that this initial increase is temporary. It's similar to when you first take up exercise and your muscles are sore because you're using them in unfamiliar ways. As the movements become more familiar, the soreness goes away. Similarly, with time the discomfort associated with noticing anxiety decreases.

Also, you will find that paying closer attention to your anxiety helps you notice responses earlier in the spiral, when they are not as intense or distressing.

Finally, we're asking you to notice your anxiety in a new and different way. People often hypervigilantly scan for signs of anxiety, either to brace for the threats to come or to chastise themselves for having an unwanted response. As you monitor your experience, try to bring a curious, observing stance to noticing your anxiety. The goal is to observe and notice the full range of reactions, not to judge or control them. Over time this new way of relating to your anxiety will lead to these signs being less alarming and overwhelming.

Problems Associated with Different Anxiety Disorders

GENERALIZED ANXIETY DISORDER

- Chronic worry about a number of different events.
- Muscle tension and other physical symptoms.
- No clear target of fear, but worry can be used to avoid pain related to important areas of living.

OBSESSIVE–COMPULSIVE DISORDER

- Frequent consuming, unwanted, frightening thoughts or images that are stronger and more intense than worry (e.g., having the strong sense that you forgot to turn off the space heater, ran someone over, or contracted a deadly virus).
  - Habits that take up a lot of time but seem necessary to prevent potential disasters, such as repeating certain phrases over and over in your mind, carefully lining objects up in a certain way, or following strict rules about how to clean.
- Target of fear is unwanted thoughts, images, or urges.

PANIC DISORDER

- Unexpected panic attacks—abrupt surges of intense fear or dread accompanied by strong physical sensations.
- Worry about what the attacks mean about one's health, safety, and well-being and fear of more in the future.
- Target of fear is bodily sensations.
- Sometimes accompanied by *agoraphobia,* which involves avoiding places from which it would be tough to escape or get help if a panic attack occurred.

POSTTRAUMATIC STRESS DISORDER

- Develops after someone is exposed to a terrifying, dangerous event that may have made the person feel powerless or victimized.
- Memories of the event are constantly recurring out of the blue, in

dreams or in response to reminders of the event. These memories are accompanied by intense fear and a desire to escape.

- A tendency to avoid reminders of events or one's own thoughts and feelings about the event, as well as feelings of diminished interest in things or detachment from other people.
- Chronic feelings of being keyed up or on edge.
- Target of fear is reminders of traumatic event, both internal (e.g., memories and feelings) and external (e.g., sights and sounds).

SOCIAL ANXIETY DISORDER OR SOCIAL PHOBIA

- Anxiety and self-consciousness in social situations.
  - Can be a specific situation (e.g., public speaking) or more general.
- Concerned about being negatively evaluated and judged by others.
- Target of fear is everyday social situations.

SPECIFIC PHOBIA

- Distressing and/or impairing fear of a specific object or situation (e.g., spiders or dogs, thunder and lightning, certain medical procedures, heights).
- Target of fear is individualized.

2

how is anxiety getting in your way?

Peter pauses on the landing to catch his breath after climbing five flights of stairs. Taking the elevator up to his office would be a lot easier, but he just can't torture himself that way. Most mornings the elevator is packed with his coworkers, chatting among themselves about sports, the weather, shows they watched on TV, and plans for the weekend. Everyone seems to join in so easily, but Peter dreads the thought of trying to make small talk.

Monday mornings are the worst. For a while Peter tried riding the elevator. Standing in the corner, pressed up against the wall, he kept his eyes on the floor, hoping to blend in with the crowd. But about 3 weeks ago Joe, a large, friendly guy from the sales department, attempted to include Peter in the conversation. With a booming voice Joe asked, "What about you, Pete? What did you do this weekend?" Peter was completely thrown by the attention. He felt everyone stare, scrutinizing him like he was a specimen under a microscope. Peter's mind went blank, and his mouth felt like it was stuffed with cotton. The seconds passed like hours until Joe finally let him off the hook with a pat on the back and a laugh, "That's all right, sport, my weekend was pretty boring too." The crowd burst into laughter as Peter hurried off the elevator and darted into the bathroom, where he remained until he heard the hallway clear. Now he just sticks to the back stairwell, hoping to avoid scrutiny.

"What was I supposed to say?" Peter wonders, now replaying the embarrassing moment in his mind. "I spent the weekend holed up in my apartment alone, watching TV, like I always do. Who is going to hang out with a freak like me who can't even carry on a 2-minute conversation without turning red and stuttering? I am 25, never had a girlfriend, and never will. Worked my ass off to earn my MBA, and I am stuck in this dead-end job because I am too afraid to venture out of my cubicle. What a total and complete failure."

Selena glances at the clock, surprised that only 5 minutes have elapsed since she last checked. A full 4 hours before her shift is up, and she is not sure she can make it through the next 30 minutes. She feels a sticky hand on her shoulder as Jacob, clutching a toy truck in his hand, steadies himself from the rocky journey across the room and then plops down beside her on the carpet. "You make a bridge so I can crash," he insists, and she stacks the blocks for what seems like the hundredth time that day. Jacob beams with pride as the blocks tumble down from the force of the truck and joyfully demands, "Again." Selena halfheartedly cooperates, pre-occupied with self-critical thoughts. "I can't believe I turned down the opportunity to teach middle school science for this job. What a loser I am. I am ruining my life. Everyone else I graduated with is starting out their careers, and I am just stuck."

Just a few months earlier Selena had thought the preschool position would be perfect for her. It seemed like a low-pressure way to stay in the field of education while she worked on trying to man-age her fear of public speaking. Selena hadn't realized how much she would miss designing creative lab activities aimed at capturing the curious minds of eighth-grade students. When she first accepted the position, she vowed she would use her free time wisely. Free from the pressures and academic challenges of running her own classroom, Selena believed she would have ample time to devote to self-improvement. She would spend her evenings reading scien-

tific journals, developing lesson plans, and working on her fears of public speaking. But this job seemed to be sucking the life out of her. She had no energy or motivation to do anything after work except eat her dinner on the couch, aimlessly surfing the channels for some show that could hold her attention.

Jacob destroys his last bridge, toddles over, and collapses onto Selena's lap, exhausted from his efforts. She shifts her weight to accommodate him and steals another glance at the clock as she resigns herself to the fact that her life, just like the clock, seems to be stalled.

Often when we think about our struggle with fear and anxiety we focus on our emotional responses. We vigilantly watch for signs that we might become anxious and search for ways to control our feelings. Struggling with anxiety is time-consuming, stressful, and exhausting. It can easily become the focus of our daily lives and can take a toll in many different ways.

Sometimes the choices we make to avoid emotions are clear, and the impact on our lives is obvious. But anxiety can also more subtly nudge us away from the things that matter most, gradually eroding our sense of connection and fulfillment. Bringing a new awareness—mindfulness—to all the concessions and compromises we make is a critical first step toward reclaiming our lives.

The Cost of Choosing to Avoid Anxiety

Behavioral avoidance—acting in ways that remove us from anxiety-provoking situations—is a key component of fear and anxiety. When we imagine that a situation or activity will bring potential threat, we may choose to **avoid** the situation. If we find ourselves afraid or anxious, we may try a number of strategies to **escape**. Or, when faced with overpowering emotions, we may **freeze** and remain immobilized or stuck in hopes that the threat or stressor will pass.

Clearly, these moves are consistent with our evolutionary instinct toward self-protection. But they also may reflect beliefs we hold about improving the quality of our lives. It is common sense to assume that avoiding people, places, and activities that could elicit fear (or even sadness or anger) will keep us safe and calm. And isn't achieving a calm and peaceful state the best way to succeed in life?

One of the trickiest things about escaping the struggle with anxiety and reclaiming one's life is reexamining that assumption. The belief that overcoming fear and doubt is the key to successful living seems logical. But following that logic may be the very thing keeping us trapped. One significant step out of that trap is to carefully and objectively observe the costs and benefits of trying to design an anxiety-free life.

Both Peter and Selena recognize that they have given up valuable opportunities in an attempt to keep anxiety at bay. Selena made a conscious decision to accept a much less appealing job in the hopes of minimizing the stress and anxiety in her life. Peter's prime directive is to avoid social interactions. He knows from experience that uncomfortable physical sensations, thoughts about his shortcomings and failures, and difficult emotions arise whenever he is around others. And so Peter's moment-to-moment choices about how to engage in his life are based on whether an action is likely to elicit fear. He leaves his building 10 minutes earlier than necessary to avoid bumping into his neighbor. He avoids eye contact, preventing anyone from trying to strike up a conversation. Peter takes his lunch to work every day so he has an

> *What are the real costs and benefits of trying to craft an anxiety-free life?*

excuse available if his coworkers invite him out. He volunteers for the most mundane and undesirable tasks when working on a group project to ensure he can work alone. He screens all of his phone calls to avoid invitations.

Both Selena and Peter believe that avoiding anxiety-provoking situations should make their lives easier, more stress free, and ultimately richer and fuller. But to move forward, both will need to acknowledge two critically important points. Their pain and suffering does not seem to be eased by avoidance. Indeed, avoidance comes with some significant costs.

Peter is sexually attracted to women, yet he doesn't talk to women; in fact, he has never been on a date. He avoids women because he doesn't want to put himself through the torture of feeling uncomfortable or being evaluated. Unfortunately, avoiding women has not protected Peter from discomfort and distress. He constantly berates himself for the choices he makes. He feels anxious and depressed much of the time.

He evaluates himself relentlessly and concludes he is worthless. On top of all this, Peter is lonely. He wants to feel connected with someone, to develop an intimate relationship. His choice to avoid social situations in the name of self-protection has clearly backfired. But rather than questioning the assumption that avoiding fear will enhance his life, or considering pursuing a relationship despite his fears and doubts, Peter remains committed to his course of action. Rather than recognizing that avoidance isn't working and exploring other strategies to enhance his quality of life, Peter simply blames himself for failing.

Similarly, Selena believed taking a less stressful job would allow her to prepare for the future. She wanted to resolve her struggle with anxiety before pursuing a position that was more consistent with her values. On the surface this decision seems reasonable. People often think they need to work through their fears, increase their self-confidence, and gain control over their emotions before accepting a challenging job or moving forward with a new relationship. The idea is that making time to address problems with anxiety in the present will pave the way for a better life in the future. Unfortunately, Selena is starting to notice that putting her life on hold while she focuses on self-improvement is not working as well as she thought it would. The day-to-day, moment-to-moment experience of spending her time on tasks she finds unsatisfying is draining and painful. She is depressed by the limited opportunities she has to engage in challenging and personally meaningful activities. And since she assumed the choice to delay teaching middle school science was the best strategy for directly addressing her fears, Selena is beginning to worry she might never be able to overcome her anxiety and land the job she wants. Selena feels like a helpless bystander in her own life.

EXERCISE **A first look at how anxiety limits our choices**

Can you identify choices you have made at *work*, in your *relationships* (family, friendships, partners), and in *community or leisure activities* that likely were driven by the desire to avoid fear or anxiety? Are there opportunities you would not pursue in any of these domains because of your fears? Consider jotting down in a notebook any thoughts that come to your mind about the ways in which you may be avoiding people, places, or activities because of fear or anxiety. We continue to explore this question in the remaining chapters; often it is very challenging to notice how avoidance has become part of our lives. Keep adding to this list as you notice evidence of avoidance in your life.

Avoiding One Thing or Just Choosing Something Else?

Vivian hasn't set foot in a shopping mall in at least 10 years. When her daughter Margaret was a baby, Vivian and her friends would meet at the food court every Wednesday for some window-shopping and a chance to catch up while the babies napped in their strollers. Then one Saturday afternoon Vivian ran out alone for a quick shopping trip. She needed to pick up a wedding gift, and the bride was registered at a home-goods store located in the center of the mall. Vivian was trying to hurry back home before the baby woke up from her nap because she was using a brand-new babysitter. She stood at the register impatiently checking her watch while the salesperson put the finishing touches on the gift-wrapped package. All of a sudden, Vivian felt blindsided by a rush of intense fear and dread. Her heart pounded in her chest, she felt her throat tighten, and she began to hyperventilate. Lightheaded and dizzy, Vivian bolted from the store, trying to escape the mall. She desperately needed fresh air, but as she searched for an exit Vivian became disoriented and confused. As she blindly rushed through the maze of a large department store, Vivian felt her legs buckle underneath her and she fell to the floor. A store employee hurried to her aid and called the paramedics. At the emergency room, after a battery of tests, Vivian was told she had experienced a panic attack.

Vivian tried to go back to the mall a few times, always accompanied by a trusted friend or family member. But each time she saw the sprawl of buildings looming in the distance, she turned around and headed home. That first Christmas Vivian did all her shopping online. She was painfully aware of missing out on many holiday traditions. Vivian's husband took Margaret to the mall to sit on Santa's lap. Vivian's friends went window-shopping without her.

Over the past 10 years Vivian has become quite a savvy Internet shopper. She receives notifications whenever an item on her wish list goes on sale, and she has bookmarked more than 25 sites that offer online coupons to her favorite stores. Vivian scorns friends and family members who still shop at malls. Why would anyone fight the crowds and pay top price for an off-the-rack outfit that everyone else will be wearing? Vivian can find one-of-a-kind items, in the comfort of her own home, at her convenience.

Vivian has been a Web shopper for so long that she considers it a preference rather than an avoidance behavior. She no longer associates her strong negative feelings about the mall with her fear of having a panic attack. Certainly, there are plenty of people who don't like going to the mall, and avoiding it doesn't seem to have any obvious negative consequences. But recently Vivian reluctantly turned down an invitation from her neighbor Rita to join a group of friends for a Sunday morning power walk through the mall. Rita was new to the neighborhood, but she and Vivian had recently swapped parenting stories and shared some laughs over coffee about how that last 10 pounds of baby weight can hang around long after the baby reaches adolescence. Vivian could see the disappointment and confusion in Rita's face when she turned down the invitation without explanation.

By all measures, it seems as though Sloane lives life to the fullest. She is somewhat quiet and reserved, preferring to keep her history private from most of her coworkers or acquaintances. But even if they knew about the struggle she faced with anxiety after being date-raped in college, most would agree she seems fully recovered.

Extremely successful in her career as a research scientist for a major pharmaceutical company, Sloane travels extensively, is a regular patron of the arts, and enjoys exploring new restaurants with her best friend and sister, Margie. Sloane finds her work extremely fulfilling and satisfying. She enjoys presenting her research at conferences and networking with scientists in her field. She also finds consulting with physicians about their most complex cases extremely satisfying.

Although Sloane lives alone in a tastefully decorated brown-stone in the city, she spends many weekends and most holidays with her sister, Margie, brother-in-law, Steve, and their children. Sloane is a fabulous aunt who always makes time for stuffed-animal tea parties, fort building, and bedtime stories with her nieces and nephew. But Sloane has no desire to become a parent herself. Nor is she interested in pursuing an intimate relationship. Although her family and colleagues have tried on occasion to set her up on a date, Sloane insists she is perfectly content and complete without a partner. She scoffs at those who think a woman needs a partner to feel complete. Her practiced response is so convincing that even Sloane herself has come to believe it. But on the rare occasion that she is alone in her apartment for more than a few days, her thoughts freed from the endless challenges of work, Sloane becomes aware of a profound sense of loneliness that is always with her, usually residing just outside of her attention.

Sloane avoids any situation in which she feels vulnerable or is reminded of the rape in an attempt to keep her anxiety at bay. When she was younger she tried dating, but she found that a gentle caress on her back or even the smell of cologne was enough to bring memories of the rape flooding back. Sloane chose to surround herself with a fortress of family members she knew she could trust, to immerse herself in her career, and to avoid taking any chances with new relationships. This choice has cost her the opportunity to develop new friends and deeply connect with a life partner.

Many of us are acutely aware of the sacrifices we make to avoid anxiety. But over time anxiety responses, including behavioral avoidance, can become so habitual that they happen outside of our awareness. Just like we might mindlessly polish off a bag of popcorn while engrossed in a movie, without much thought or consideration, we might turn down an invitation for lunch, pass up an opportunity at work, or go out of our way to avoid a neighbor to avoid possible discomfort. And the more frequently we choose to act on avoidance, the less aware we become of that pattern.

A common reaction to hearing about Vivian, Sloane, and others with similar stories is to wonder about the difference between behavioral avoidance and preference. After all, many of us detest shopping at the mall, and certainly there is nothing wrong with choosing to remain single. Making this distinction is tricky, and it requires a heightened sense of personal awareness, the kind of mindful awareness we hope to help you cultivate through this book.

The "Turning toward Your Emotions" exercise introduced at the end of Chapter 1 can help you increase your awareness of when you're acting on a true preference and when you're trying to avoid an anxiety-raising situation. Although most of us can pretty easily list situations or activities that make us nervous, our emotional responses are extremely complex and, unless we are really paying attention, we can miss more subtle cues of anxiety. We present new exercises throughout this book to help you develop awareness of these subtleties and determine when your actions are based on avoidance rather than preference.

For example, one behavioral response to fear-eliciting threat cues is "fight." Sloane gets extremely angry and irritated when a family member asks her about whether she is dating. Often she launches into a speech about female stereotypes, accusing the speaker of believing that women cannot be fulfilled without the experience of motherhood. Sloane also feels anxious when this topic comes up, but she is not usually tuned in to this emotion. Anger and anxiety share so many signs—increased heart rate, a flushed sensation, muscle tension—that it can be difficult to tease them apart. Also, anger and anxiety have a reciprocal relationship. As anger increases, anxiety tends to decrease. A slight threat, a flutter of vulnerability, a hint of anxiety can automatically cue feelings of anger that leave Sloane feeling powerful and strong rather than weak and frightened. And because this response occurs so automatically, she is unaware of the process. If Sloane begins to turn toward her emotions and watches them unfold, she may recognize anxiety along with anger and become more conscious of her avoidance.

Going through the Motions: Subtle Avoidance of Painful Internal States

"Daddy, it's your turn," Hannah shouts impatiently as she sweeps her pile of checkers onto the floor and abruptly pushes her chair back from the table. "I quit. I don't like playing with you—it's no fun." The outburst startles Eric, who was engrossed in thoughts

about how to manage an upcoming meeting with his boss. His attention shifts back to the present moment just in time for him to watch Hannah stumble up the stairs to her bedroom, her eyes brimming with tears of frustration. Eric lets out a heavy sigh and gingerly massages his temple to defend against the tension headache that is building in intensity. If he doesn't work this conflict out with his 8-year-old daughter, all hell will break loose when his wife, Lori, gets home.

Last weekend he and Lori had a big blowout about Eric's job and the toll it was taking on the family. Eric had tried to defend himself, arguing that he was the first to leave the office every day despite enormous pressures to stay and work late into the evening. "What's the point?" Lori responded, her voice dripping with contempt. "From the moment you set foot in the house until you pass out on the couch, you are glued to your BlackBerry. Your idea of spending quality time with Hannah is sitting next to her while she watches 'SpongeBob' and you check your e-mail. And I can't remember the last time you actually made it upstairs to sleep in your own bed. Just 5 more minutes, you promise every night, but in the morning, chances are I will find you asleep on the couch, the laptop screen glowing with whatever document you were working on when you finally passed out."

Deep down, Eric recognized that Lori was right, but he felt trapped between a rock and a hard place. The expectations and pressure on him at work were significant, but lately he spent much of his time in the office ruminating about his shortcomings as a husband and father and worrying about whether Lori would leave him. During these episodes he would become paralyzed with fear, which was making him fall further and further behind at work. Yet when he was home, his mind would become overwhelmed with worries about losing his job, and he felt compelled to tie up the loose ends of the day. After the fight Eric had resolved to try harder at work and at home, but he felt hopeless, like he was a spectator in his own life, watching himself just going through the motions.

Filled with guilt and remorse, Eric trudges up the stairs toward his daughter's bedroom in an attempt to restore peace. "Anyone want to join me for some ice cream and a movie?" he asks with false cheer. Hannah nods excitedly and springs from her bed, her

mood lifted at the thought of receiving two treats usually limited to
special occasions. "Don't tell Mommy; it will be our secret," Eric
nearly pleads. A temporary relief washes over him as they snuggle
together on the couch in front of the television, a container of ice
cream between them. But the relief vanishes as the buzz of his
BlackBerry prompts a flood of new worries.

Most of us can easily identify people, places, or activities that we
have avoided at one time or another because of fear or anxiety. But we
might be less aware of how avoidance can influence the **quality** of our
participation in meaningful life events. On the surface it may seem like
we are diligent in managing several important life domains. We might
devote significant time and energy to our jobs, regularly socialize with
family and friends, tirelessly volunteer with a number of different groups
in the community. But careful observation sometimes reveals that we
are not fully engaged in or attentive to the activities that make up our
daily lives.

Clearly, Eric's worries about work and his family are interfering
with his effectiveness as an employee, spouse, and father. They are
also eroding his overall quality of life, his sense of enjoyment, satisfaction, and purpose. Eric is frustrated because the efforts he is making to
improve his performance at work and to connect with his family have
not been effective. His boss is growing concerned because Eric continues to leave the office at 5:00 P.M. each day even as he falls further and
further behind on his work. Lori is exasperated by the fact that Eric
seems to be prioritizing his work over his family. A much closer examination of Eric's anxiety and avoidance are needed to better understand
his struggle.

Eric sprints from the bus stop toward his office, hoping to slip behind
his desk before his boss notices that Eric is late again. Of course
the reason he is late is that he didn't fall asleep until almost 2:00
A.M. because he was up worrying about the fourth-quarter report
that is due by the end of the day. Eric fell asleep on the couch, and
Lori was in the shower when his alarm went off. By the time she
finished up in the bathroom and realized that Eric was still asleep
on the couch, he had already missed his usual bus.

The receptionist glances meaningfully at the clock as Eric
hurries to his cubicle. He signs in to his e-mail and is immediately

bombarded with messages, one from his boss marked as high prior-ity. Eric can feel himself break out in a sweat, and his heart begins to pound. He knows that he should read the message immediately, but he feels lightheaded and dizzy. Instead, Eric stands up and heads to the men's room, fighting an urge to run out of the build-ing. As he splashes cold water onto his face, Eric's thoughts return to his family. He feels guilty about letting Hannah watch a movie because Lori is always preaching about the negative effects of tele-vision on children. Eric returns to his desk, minimizes his inbox, and begins to search the Internet for articles on the link between television viewing habits and academic achievement. Eric quickly becomes absorbed by the debate and spends an hour researching the topic. As he reads he begins to worry about whether he is sav-ing enough for Hannah's college education. Eric signs in to his 401K account to check his balance and read about loan options.

Right around noon Eric is startled by the ringing of his phone. He checks his caller ID and lets the call roll over to voice mail. Lori is calling to remind him that he promised to be home early and to join her at Hannah's school play, without his BlackBerry. Eric silently resolves to work on his report so he can leave at the strike of 5:00. He spends the remaining hours of the afternoon pulling together a draft, but his efforts are halfhearted. Eric knows that it will be impossible to produce quality work in the time he has. He hopes his boss will understand that Eric had to attend Hannah's school event.

Eric meets Lori outside of the auditorium, and together they quickly weave through the crowd to get a seat in the front. Eric is filled with overwhelming pride as he watches Hannah perform. Lori reaches for his hand and squeezes it, a simple gesture that con-veys both love and forgiveness. For a moment Eric feels at peace as he considers how lucky he is to have such a wonderful family. But these warm, positive feelings quickly fade as he considers how close he is to losing them both. Eric feels an intense surge of fear as he realizes that Lori will likely leave him unless he is able to set firm boundaries between his work and home life. With a jolt he remembers that he never read the e-mail from his boss. For the remainder of the performance, Eric is distracted by thinking about all of the possible issues that his boss could have raised in the e-mail message.

At first glance, it is hard to see any avoidance in Eric's behavior. He deeply values both his work and his family, and he is consumed by thoughts and worries about both life domains. But closer observation suggests a different, more subtle form of avoidance may be present. Specifically, Eric often worries about possible, but not imminent, negative outcomes as a way to avoid the immediate experience of intense fear. For example, when Eric is confronted with a task at work that cues fear, he worries about his family as a way to distract himself and manage his emotions. Although worrying is still associated with a negative mood state, it dampens the intense panic that was building in response to the more immediate work-related threat. Similarly, general worry about work distracts Eric from the intense fear and sadness of contemplating the loss of his family. Engaging in worry about a possible future event rather than experiencing intense emotion in response to a current situation is sort of a "lesser of two evils" form of avoidance. Noticing it when it happens requires letting go of preconceived notions and assumptions about the nature of anxiety and worry and carefully observing responses as a situation unfolds.

If Eric were to bring mindfulness to his current struggles, several changes would be possible. First, he would recognize when his attention was being pulled away from the present moment, and he would have the skills needed to refocus on the present moment. Eric would also be able to see how worrying about his family while at work and about work while with his family is driven by his

> *Mindfulness can reveal avoidance ... and do a lot more to help you manage anxiety.*

desire to live in accordance with his values in both of these domains. On the other hand, mindfulness would give Eric the clarity to recognize that worrying is actually a fairly ineffective way of demonstrating his commitment to these life areas. Instead, Eric would use mindfulness skills to bring compassion to the difficulty of balancing work and home and create a space in which he could devote his full energy and attention to his family when he is with them and to his work when he is at work. Finally, mindfulness would allow Eric to feel effective and derive satisfaction from his actions in both domains, rather than feeling confused and helpless.

Annie leans forward in her seat, fingers poised above the keyboard of her laptop, eyes fixed on the board. Although her body is situ-

ated in a classroom, her mind is replaying an earlier conversation with her long-term boyfriend, David. What had started as a discussion about their weekend plans had devolved into a bitter argument. "It was completely irresponsible of David to invite people over for dinner," Annie fumed to herself. "Finals are coming up, and we have to ace these exams if we want to get into graduate school. Plus, we haven't cleaned the apartment or done laundry at all in the last week. It would be so embarrassing if anyone saw what a wreck the place is. We just don't have the time this weekend to socialize with anyone," Annie concluded. But David was so irrational and irresponsible. He couldn't see that canceling the plans was the most rational course of action. When Annie tried to explain her logic, David just shook his head and muttered, "What happened to you? It's like you don't even know how to have fun anymore."

Back in the classroom, the professor interrupts the lecture to hand back a graded assignment. As he shuffles up and down the aisle, Annie studies the photo background on her desktop—a picture of her and David during their last vacation. She can't help noticing how young they both look, the silly grin plastered on her face as she watches David mug for the camera. Annie replays the morning's argument over and over in her mind. She has always been responsible and hard-working. But lately it does seem like she is just going through the motions, completing chore after chore, trying to keep everything perfect. Annie is startled by the realization that, in her quest to remain focused and on track, she may be jeopardizing the very things that matter most to her.

As a high school student things had come easily for Annie. She did well in school, had a close-knit circle of friends, and had a boyfriend on whom she could rely. Things changed when she went to college. No longer a big fish in a small pond, Annie felt intimidated by her classmates and had difficulty developing new friendships. She began to fear that David would realize that Annie was not particularly special or unique and break up with her to pursue a different relationship.

For the first time in her life, Annie felt extremely vulnerable and unsure about her place in the world and began to worry about her future. The sadness, fear, and doubt she was suddenly confronted with frightened her, and she did not allow herself to fully *experience these responses to her new situation. As a way to keep her fears about the future somewhat contained, Annie began to worry incessantly about minor matters. Annie's apartment needed to be kept neat and clean at all times. She could not tolerate being late for classes or appointments. Every homework assignment, quiz, test, or paper had to be completed perfectly. Annie even began to approach her social life and leisure activities with the same perspective. In an attempt to remain popular, Annie tried to schedule lunch with a classmate at least once a week. She and David went to the movies or dinner with another couple at least once a month. Although Annie enjoyed outdoor activities such as hiking and skiing, she allowed herself only one excursion a month.*

Focusing on these small, achievable goals felt manageable to Annie and gave her a sense of control. Unfortunately, it also distracted her from the simple pleasures of living from moment to moment, enjoying the challenges inherent in college, and appreciating her relationships. Annie was thriving academically. She remained a serious, responsible student, was active in a variety of campus organizations, and generously volunteered her time at a local hospital. She had a long-term relationship with someone who cared deeply about her. But avoiding the pain of feeling vulnerable and frightened was subtly leaching the enjoyment out of what seemed on the surface to be a full, busy, meaningful life. Avoidance often comes at a cost.

> *Avoidance comes at a cost that we may not notice without mindfulness.*

Habitual Avoidance:
Restrictive Instead of Protective

Fear is a natural response to an immediate perceived threat. Avoidance is a behavioral tendency aimed at reducing fear, dodging threat, and maximizing our chances of survival. Unfortunately, without much thought or effort on our part, efforts to avoid fear and pain can develop into habits and preferences that have an impact on every aspect of our lives. When we struggle with anxiety, choices about how we spend our time, where we invest our energy, and whom we open up to can be driven more by our attempts to avoid fear and vulnerability than by our desire to engage in meaningful and valued activities.

It is sometimes easier to notice how avoidance affects the big decisions in life: which career we pursue (a position in accounting rather than sales, for example); whether we commit to or terminate a relationship; how we spend our free time (taking up a solitary activity like long-distance running vs. volunteering at a church). We often pay less attention to the subtle ways avoidance nudges us to respond moment by moment to the choices that arise. Should I have a glass of water or a soda? Do I sleep in today or get up early and go for a run? Should I call a friend tonight or watch TV? Should I stay at work and finish this project or visit my grandfather in the nursing home? Do I confront my partner or let the issue go? Although we pay them less attention, these moment-by-moment choices considerably affect our quality of life.

> *Tianna thinks about the importance of exercising almost every day. Several mornings a week as she lies in bed she thinks about ways she might incorporate more physical activity into her day. Several of her friends have regular exercise routines; maybe she could call one of them and ask if she could tag along at the next cycling class. She has also discussed taking a class at the Y with her partner, Roy. She thinks about how that would both bring them closer and help them engage in a healthier lifestyle. Her kids have a Wii, and she has tried playing Wii Fit and Dance, Dance Revolution a few times. Maybe scheduling a regularly occurring family Wii night would be an easy way to fit exercise into her busy life.*
>
> *But when Tianna sees some of her friends at the corner dropping their kids off at the bus stop, her fear of intruding on them holds her back from asking about the cycling class. Plus, they have been exercising for a while and she could never catch up. As usual, Tianna's day at the office is busy and stressful. In an attempt to avoid any conflict with her boss, she stays at work until she finishes the last of a pile of expense reports and misses her usual train home. As she runs to the station so as not to miss the next train, Tianna calls Roy to ask if he will pick up some fast food on the way home. There is no time tonight for a healthy, home-cooked meal. Tianna is met by a jumble of activity when she steps into her house. Apparently, her eldest daughter is responsible for bringing baked goods to*

her club meeting the next day, and her son put off studying for his test because he really needs Tianna's help. Swiftly and efficiently, Tianna begins whipping up a batch of brownies while quizzing her son on the different empires of Mesopotamia. Although she licks the pan along the way, she is still starving when Roy hits the door, and she digs into one of the warm bags he drops on the counter and fishes out a handful of salty fries. After the kids are taken care of, the cats fed, and the laundry pushed along, Tianna collapses on the couch for a little restorative "me" time. She feels too exhausted to even consider working out and instead flips on the television to help her wind down. The next morning as she contemplates how to lead a healthier lifestyle she concludes that the situation is hopeless and out of her control.

Tianna is unaware of the multitude of small choices she made that culminated in her choice not to exercise. The decision not to bring up cycling at the bus stop on one particular day seemed insignificant in the moment. She didn't consider leaving work at the regular time because she automatically defers to her boss's requests to avoid his disapproval. Tianna does not recognize that she places the preferences of her children before her own needs without thought or hesitation. She did not consider how food choices would affect her physical and psychological motivation. Tianna made several small in-the-moment choices aimed at avoiding anxiety and reducing stress. But at the time she didn't see most of them as choices, nor did she connect them with her desire to live healthily.

In addition to severely limiting our choices and activities, avoidance can prevent us from acting effectively in a situation. Eric's unwillingness to directly experience the fear he would feel if he fully engaged in his work is threatening both his job security and his marriage. Annie's rigid attempts to be perfect, which she hopes will keep her safe and loved, are also backfiring, creating conflict and distance in the very relationship she hopes to keep. When we are focused on threat, and all of our efforts are aimed at avoiding fear and pain, we are less tuned in to the consequences of our behavior. We can miss the

> *Making lots of little choices without being aware of trying to avoid anxiety can add up to big choices we never thought we made.*

essential clues that remind us that a new or different response is needed. Avoidance can keep us stuck, using ineffective strategies in an attempt to improve our lives.

EXERCISE **A closer look at avoidance and the ways it may be holding you back**

This exercise involves freely expressing your deepest thoughts and emotions about the ways in which anxiety and avoidance may be preventing you from having the life you desire.

We would like you to explore four different topics (described below) in a writing exercise. You should limit your writing to one topic per day so that you have time to really focus on each exercise.

Each day, choose a time when you can devote an uninterrupted 20 minutes to the exercise (we recommend setting a timer). Choose a location that is private and where you feel comfortable and safe exploring your deepest and most honest emotions.

Each day, keep in mind a few important topics we have discussed:

- Mindfully approaching this exercise involves:
  - Turning toward something that we would usually avoid.
  - Taking a fresh look at a familiar response (approaching it with curiosity).
  - Bringing gentle self-compassion to your responses, rather than harsh criticism (this takes practice and we will work on it together; for now just try to respond to yourself with kindness as best you can).
- Avoidance includes:
  - Making obvious choices to avoid people, places, and activities that elicit fear.
  - Subtle changes in behavior that are sometimes disguised as preferences.
  - Going through the motions and not truly engaging in important activities.
  - Making little choices and compromises to reduce distress without being fully aware of your actions and their consequences.

As you write, try to allow yourself to experience your thoughts and feelings as completely as you can. If you can't think of what to write next, repeat the same thing until something new comes to you. Be sure to write for the entire 20 minutes. Don't be concerned with spelling, punctuation, or grammar; just express whatever comes to mind.

DAY 1

Please write about how you think your anxiety and worry might be interfering with your relationships (family, friends, partner, etc.). Here are some questions to consider to get you started:

- What are some things that you do when you are anxious that affect your relationships?
- How do your anxiety and worry hold you back in relationships?
- What do you need from others in your life? What do you want to give to others? What gets in the way of asking for what you need and giving what you want to give?
- Do you make choices in your relationships that are driven by avoidance?
- Are you present and engaged when you are with others?

DAY 2

Please write about how you think your anxiety and worry might be interfering with your work, education or training, or your family/ household management if you are a stay-at-home parent. You might think about these questions:

- What are some things that you do when anxious that affect your job/studies?
- How do anxiety and worry hold you back in your work/schooling?
- Are there changes that you would like to make in this area of your life?
- Do you make choices in your work/studies/household management that are driven by avoidance?
- Are you present and engaged when working, studying, or managing your household?

DAY 3

Please write about how you think your anxiety and worry interfere with your ability to take care of yourself, have fun, and/or get involved with your community. For example:

- What are some activities in these areas that you would like to spend more time doing?
- How do your anxiety and worry hold you back?
- Do you make choices about your leisure or community-based activities that are driven by avoidance?
- Are you present and engaged when participating in leisure or community-based activities?

DAY 4

This is your last day of writing, so take some time to reflect on what came up for you over the last few days as you allowed yourself to focus on the issues raised in the first three writing assignments. Have you noticed any important areas that need more attention? Have you noticed activities or situations that you avoid because of your anxiety in any areas of your life? Feel free to write about whatever comes up for you about these three areas of living.

3

changing your relationship
with anxiety

EMBARKING ON A NEW PATH

Despite the fact that fear and anxiety are helpful emotions experienced by all humans, many of us are locked in a chronic struggle with these states. Avoiding situations and activities that could elicit anxiety seems like a way to restore peace and balance to our lives. Unfortunately, this strategy doesn't seem to relieve distress significantly, and it keeps us from fully engaging in life.

As you saw in the stories told in Chapter 2, the struggle with anxiety can take a toll on our physical and emotional well-being, cause conflict in our relationships, and diminish the overall quality of our lives. Struggling with anxiety keeps Eric from fully paying attention to either his work or his family, and he's feeling the fallout in both arenas. Tianna avoids so many of her moment-to-moment experiences to eliminate anxiety—from asking friends if she can join their exercise group to confronting her boss about having to miss deadlines—that she has no idea how these choices have contributed to her apparent inability to start getting in shape. Anxiety about the future and her recent feelings of vulnerability are keeping Annie from pursuing and enjoying what she values most in life.

The goal of this book is to demonstrate how you can use mindfulness to disengage from your struggle with anxiety and fully participate in your life. Mindfulness (described more fully in the next chapter) is a skill that all humans already possess. But, as with every other skill, the more you practice it, the easier it is to use. In this chapter you'll learn how mindfulness practice can directly affect three major consequences of struggling with anxiety:

• To escape our fears, we often restrict or narrow our attention, and this lack of flexible attention makes it difficult to make informed choices. Mindfulness involves paying attention in a unique way. When we are mindful we notice where our attention is focused, and we may choose to shift or expand our attention. The quality of attention in mindfulness is also special. As mentioned earlier, it involves taking a fresh look at a familiar response—bringing a gentle curiosity and compassion to our experiences.

• Another way we avoid anxiety and stress is to try to opt out of our experience—the thoughts, emotions, sensations, and all the rest—which can cause us to throw out the proverbial baby with the bathwater. Being mindful allows us to appreciate and participate in all aspects of our lives, even the more difficult and painful moments. We can use this skill to be more effective and present in our everyday activities.

• Eliminating anxiety can become an all-consuming effort, leaving us little time for experiencing the joy and fulfillment of whatever we find meaningful in daily life. Mindfulness encourages us to enjoy being fully engaged in life and to keep pursuing what matters most.

Problem 1: Struggles with Anxiety Interfere with Attention

Keisha watches the seconds tick by on the clock hanging at the front of the lecture hall. According to her calculations, there is time for only two more student presentations, and the odds are 1 to 5 that she will be chosen to go today. Keisha panics at the dryness in her mouth and debates whether she should take a drink from her water bottle now or conserve the water in case she is called on to present. Cautiously, she reaches out toward the bottle to sneak a sip and notices with despair that her hand is shaking. Keisha scans the room to see if there is anything she can use to prop up her notes

when she is standing at the front of the class. Her initial plan had
been to hold the note cards in her hand, but her shakiness would
be too visible. Keisha glances down at her note cards; maybe she
should run through the presentation in her head just in case. But
looking at the words swimming on the page makes her more anxious, so she flips the stack of cards over and looks away.

She knows she should pay attention to the current presenter,
but Keisha is absorbed in her own thoughts. She puts hours into
reading and studying for this class every week, and she is barely
pulling off a C average. Keisha imagines the whispering, snicker-
ing, and eye-rolling that will break out as she stumbles through her
talk. None of Keisha's friends even know about her struggle with
anxiety. Her fear is limited to public speaking, and she has been
so careful to avoid classes with a presentation requirement. This
professor never assigned a project before—why couldn't he have
waited one more year before changing the syllabus? Keisha imagines the reaction of her sorority sisters when they hear about the
disastrous presentation. Her reputation for being poised and cool
under pressure will be blown completely.

Keisha is startled by the polite applause that breaks out as her
roommate Joslin gathers up her notes and makes her way back to
her seat. "How did I do?" Joslin whispers eagerly, but Keisha is too
busy trying to avoid eye contact with her professor to respond. Joslin's smile fades, and she rolls her eyes, thinking to herself, "Keisha
is so self-absorbed and stuck up. She couldn't care less about me or
my presentation."

The next student up is Andres. He and Keisha sometimes
grab a coffee in the student union after class, and she had been
thinking of inviting him to a party at her friend's apartment this
weekend. Andres flashes her a confident grin as he heads up the
aisle to the front of the class and tries to catch her eye several times
throughout the presentation. He is trying to impress her with the
depth and quality of his work. But Keisha stares ahead blankly
with a solemn look on her face that Andres misinterprets as boredom and disinterest. In reality, Keisha is frantically searching her
memory for strategies to control her anxiety. "Once in high school,
I tried picturing everyone in their underwear, but that just made
me more embarrassed," she recalls.

Somehow Keisha makes it through the rest of class, and a wave of relief washes over her when she realizes her presentation is postponed for another day. She turns to Joslin, intending to treat her to a celebratory lunch downtown, but her roommate storms away with a cold, angry expression on her face. Puzzled by her friend's response, Keisha tries to catch up with Andres. Maybe they could grab lunch at the union and she would work up the courage to invite him to the party. Andres glances her way for a moment, and Keisha smiles, but it is too late. Andres has already turned away and is walking back toward his dorm with a group of friends. Keisha feels her relief drain away, replaced by feelings of sadness and confusion as she walks across the campus alone.

Our attention is narrowed and diminished.

To increase our chances of survival in the face of danger, fear directs us to focus all of our attention on whatever threat is before us. The anxious apprehension of a future threat motivates us to continuously scan the environment for potential danger. Although this narrow and selective attention is aimed at keeping us safe, it prevents us from noticing and attending to nonthreatening parts of our experience. For example, if we are shopping at a convenience store and an armed robber storms in, our attention will be focused on his every move. The fact that we don't notice that the milk is on sale is inconsequential. But in other situations where we are afraid or anxious, missing out on the details may have more significant consequences.

In the last chapter, we considered how our preoccupation with worry and anxiety can reduce the enjoyment and pleasure we get out of our experiences. Eric clearly values his family and tries to make spending time with them a priority. Although he is physically present with his wife and daughter a fair amount of the time, because he is consumed with worry and inattentive, the relationships are strained and distant. Narrowed attention keeps Eric from fully connecting with his family.

When our attention is fixed on possible threats, we may also overlook valuable information that could help us more effectively pursue what matters most. Keisha clearly cares about others and wants their acceptance and approval. She believes that the best way to connect with others is to control her anxiety and avoid negative evaluation.

Unfortunately, Keisha's intense self-focus prevented her from noticing how her behavior affected others. Ironically, observing and responding effectively to these cues—praising Joslin for a fabulous presentation, nodding and smiling at Andres during his talk—would have provided Keisha with the very social approval and connection she was seeking. Keisha's limited awareness of her behavior and its consequences leaves her confused about the way her classmates responded. Her narrowed attention prevented her from learning from her experience. It is likely she will continue to rigidly apply the same ineffective anxiety control strategy the next time she encounters a social threat.

> Ben slams his cell phone shut and throws it across the room in anger. Once again, he has been unable to convince his brother, David, to stop drinking and check into a rehab program. No surprise, he silently fumes, David has always been thick-skulled, stubborn, and irresponsible.
>
> Ben's mother died when he and David were both just kids, and for 2 years they were shuffled from relative to relative like unwanted baggage. Finally, their father showed up and dragged them halfway across the country to live in a dingy one-bedroom apartment. Ben couldn't wait to escape that hellhole, and the day he graduated from high school he went straight to his local recruiter and enlisted in the Marine Corps. Now Ben was working on completing his graduate degree in engineering.
>
> David, on the other hand, had dropped out of school when he turned 16 and worked alongside their father at the meat-packing plant. David couldn't keep a dime in his pocket. He spent most of his money on booze, and whatever was left over he blew at the racetrack. David was the biological father of three children with two different women who were constantly taking him to court for missed child-support payments.
>
> At least once a month Ben would get on David about his dead-end life. Ben knew it was his responsibility as the older brother to set David straight. But no matter how much he yelled, screamed, and berated his brother, Ben just could not get through to David. Last week Ben had even driven all the way out to David's apartment for a face-to-face confrontation. Not only was he unsuccessful in convincing David to stop drinking; he also couldn't get his

mule-headed brother to go and see a doctor even though he had been throwing up blood for a week.

Disgusted with his failed efforts, Ben decides to head to the library to work on his school assignments. He methodically makes his way through the first problem set before noticing the tightness in his chest and the tingling, numbing sensation in his arms and legs. Ben begins to panic. Heart disease runs in his family, and he fears he is in the midst of a heart attack. He lurches toward the reference desk to ask the librarian for help and is startled by the realization that tears are streaming down his face. "What the hell is wrong with me? I must be losing my mind," he thinks in horror.

Keisha's ability to observe and respond to her environment—notably the people whom she values—was diminished by the narrowing of attention that resulted from her struggles with anxiety. But this narrowing of attention can also inhibit us from fully noticing and understanding our own internal experiences. We may recognize that we are in a bad mood or upset, but we miss important nuances involved in our emotional responding. Ben is clear that David's behavior angers him, but his narrowed attention makes him less aware of his feelings of fear, sadness, and guilt about David's health and well-being. In turn, Ben has difficulty acknowledging the grief he feels about losing his mother, accepting the profound sadness of not being able to prevent David from making harmful choices, and noticing how alone he feels without a family he can depend on. Because Ben has such a limited awareness of the complexity of the emotions he is experiencing, he is frightened and confused by their intensity.

> *Having your attention commandeered by anxiety is like focusing a telescope on the tangled brush blocking your path and failing to see the hungry lion approaching from the left or the rescuer beckoning you to safety on the right. Mindfulness gives you a wide-angle lens.*

The efficacy of Ben's actions is also limited by his restricted awareness of his emotions. Intense anger pervades all of his interactions with David, and as a result the brothers are mostly estranged. If Ben could express his vulnerability, share his fear and sadness, they might be able to share a closer bond. The confrontational strategy Ben uses to try to get through to his brother consistently backfires as David shuts down whenever he feels attacked. David might be more receptive to Ben's advice to seek treatment if he knew how frightened and sad Ben was. Yet the brothers are locked in a vicious cycle. The more concerned and hopeless Ben feels about losing his brother, the angrier he becomes. And the more he lashes out at David, the less likely it is that the two will connect.

EXERCISE **Common beliefs about anxiety**

Which of the following common beliefs about anxiety do you hold?

- "I don't like to feel anxious because I believe it is a sign of weakness."
- "I get angry with myself for feeling nervous when there is no need to be."
- "I am disappointed in myself for being so anxious."
- "I feel flawed in some way because I get anxious in situations that don't bother other people."
- "I find my anxiety overwhelming."
- "I think anxiety can be dangerous."
- "I feel defined by my anxiety."
- "Before I can move forward with my life, I have to get my anxiety under control."
- "If I were a stronger person, I could stop myself from feeling anxious."

Our attention becomes reactive and self-critical.

Our struggle with fear and anxiety arises not from any actual harm caused by the physical sensations of these emotions. It comes from our **reaction** to these emotions and the thoughts, sensations, and images that accompany them. Consider the case of Jim. Joe and Jim both have teenage daughters who recently got their licenses. Both men have concerns about their daughter's safety. At times, Joe will be sitting at his desk working on the computer and will notice worries about his daughter's well-being catching his attention. Sometimes even vivid and frightening images of her car smashed and flipped over on the side of the road pop into his mind. When these signs of anxiety surface, he acknowledges these reactions to be normal signs of being the concerned dad of a teenager. Eventually the thoughts and images pass and Joe is able to attend to other things.

> *Criticizing ourselves for feeling fear or anxiety is what hurts us—not the emotions themselves. Mindfulness can help us replace self-criticism with compassion.*

Jim also worries about his daughter's safety, but he finds these worries deeply disturbing. Jim knows it is not rational, but he has a superstitious feeling that if he imagines something terrible happening to his daughter, or experiences any doubts about her driving skills, she will be more likely to get into a crash. Jim thinks these thoughts are ridiculous and doesn't want anyone, especially his wife, to know about his concerns. His coworker, Joe, has a daughter who also just got her license. But Joe is always laughing and joking about his kids; he is not the slightest bit concerned about his daughter's driving safety. Joe's apparent cavalier attitude makes Jim feel that much worse about his own private reaction. "What the hell is wrong with me?" Jim thinks one particularly difficult day when he notices himself tearing up at the thought of losing his daughter. "A grown man crying about something that didn't even happen?" Jim thinks incredulously. "I better pull myself together before everyone starts to see how nuts I really am." Soon Jim develops the habit of drinking just a few beers each night to ease his mind. He finds that drinking calms him down enough so that he can fall asleep and push the disturbing thoughts and images out of his mind, at least for a few hours.

Jim's response to his anxiety is a pretty common one. Even though fear is a natural human response, many people are socialized to see it as a sign of weakness, irrationality, or failure. And because we often cannot see that other people are also experiencing fear and anxiety (just as Jim doesn't realize that Joe worries too), our belief that we alone are experiencing anxiety further teaches us to see it as a weakness or flaw. Because of that learning, we respond to fear and anxiety in a critical and judgmental way, viewing them as dangerous and overwhelming. Although emotions are reactions or responses to internal and external events, we feel personally responsible for our emotions and believe we should be able to control them.

We become defined by our emotional experiences.

Psychologist Steven Hayes and his colleagues have established that another uniquely human reaction to our thoughts, feelings, and sensations is to become fused with, or defined by, these experiences. In other words, rather than seeing fear as an emotion that comes and goes, we come to view it as an inherent part of our personality. Instead of acknowledging that most people occasionally have the thought "I am no good," we believe it reflects the fact that we are different or flawed in some way.

Unfortunately, all of these reactions to fear and anxiety can feed on each other, creating a cycle of anxiety that is difficult to escape. For example, Claudia sees herself as flawed because she experiences fear and anxiety in social interactions. If she is planning to attend a party, she often starts to worry about her appearance or become anxious about making small talk. These fears and worries disturb her because she sees them as unique character flaws. She is certain others don't struggle the way she does; she can tell by how at ease most people seem at parties, at least on television. Naturally, her fear brings up urges to avoid, and Claudia inevitably calls with an excuse as to why she can't make the party. Because Claudia views anxiety as an obstacle that prevents her from making and keeping friends, she becomes angry, frustrated, and hopeless whenever the emotion arises. Claudia believes she cannot be happy or live life to its fullest until she rids herself of anxious thoughts and feelings. Thus she is extremely disappointed and deflated whenever anxious symptoms arise.

> *Mindfulness can help you see that you are not your anxiety.*

Solution 1: Mindfulness Allows Us to Bring an Expanded, Compassionate Attention to Our Experience

Mindfulness practice teaches us how to focus, expand, or redirect our attention. It teaches us to recognize when our mind is pulled away from the present and toward an imagined, feared future event or an upsetting episode from the past. Cultivating this awareness allows us to return our focus to the present so that we can participate more fully in our lives. Mindfulness can help us notice the layers and nuances of our thoughts and emotions, which promotes a deeper understanding of our internal reactions and allows us to flexibly consider our options. Broadened attention also increases our awareness of the consequences of our actions and makes it easier for us to learn from our experiences.

A key feature of mindfulness is that it changes our relationship with our internal experiences. Although anxiety prompts us to turn away from uncomfortable or painful experiences, mindfulness allows us to approach them. Rather than judging some internal experiences to be acceptable or desirable and others to be unacceptable or loathsome, mindfulness involves bringing curiosity and compassion to all of our experiences. It encourages us to acknowledge that experiencing a full range of thoughts and feelings is what defines us as human.

> *It's natural to try to avoid pain, but avoiding it prevents us from understanding it and therefore dealing with it effectively.*

The more we struggle with anxiety, the more we begin to respond out of habit. Any new situation might appear threatening, and our first response is often avoidance. Mindfulness allows us to look at each situation with a fresh eye, to curiously explore our anxious reactions as if they were a novel experience, and to consider new options that were previously hidden.

Problem 2: Struggles with Anxiety Motivate Us to Avoid Our Experience

Most of us have been in some sort of relationship—with a friend, coworker, or partner—that turned sour. Let's use the example of a deteriorating relationship with an employee, Chet, to consider the stages that you pass through as the relationship dissolves. Imagine that, based on your experience, Chet is not particularly helpful or supportive. You cannot see what value Chet brings to the company; he has no special skills or talents as far as you can tell. Soon you become easily annoyed and frustrated by Chet whenever you bump into him. He seems to push all your buttons. You start to notice all the mistakes he makes, and even though you've warned him that he had better turn it around, every time you intervene, somehow things actually get worse. You can't help becoming very critical of what you view as his character flaws. As the relationship worsens, you start to avoid Chet. If you expect him to be in the break room at lunch, you eat at your desk. If you're talking with someone and he joins the conversation, you walk away. You take the long way around the office to use the bathroom because you don't want to pass Chet's desk. You strategize ways to keep him busy so that he is not available to attend your weekly staff meeting. After each unplanned encounter you spend hours fuming over his incompetence. Soon you realize your efforts to avoid Chet are actually getting in the way of your focusing on your own work because of the time and mental energy you're devoting to dealing with him. Finally, you reach your breaking point. You decide enough is enough, and you fire him. You hope you will never run into him again.

It can be challenging to end a relationship with someone, even if you no longer see his value, he pushes your buttons, and you're convinced he'll never be able to change. Unfortunately, it's impossible to end a relationship with your anxiety and other emotions, thoughts, and sensations. If you have a reactive, critical, and fused relationship with your anxiety, it makes sense that you would want to "break up." But because that's impossible, perhaps the best you can do is try to avoid your experiences at all costs.

One of the biggest struggles we have with anxiety—anxious thoughts, related emotions, sensations of tension and arousal—is that we want to avoid it. The more we struggle, the more motivated we are to use distraction, the power of positive thinking, a glass (or several) of wine, a carton of ice cream, or hours of mind-numbing reality television to try to avoid anxiety. As we discuss later in the book, unfortunately these efforts often backfire and create more distress and life interference.

Efforts to avoid our experience also contribute to the narrowed and restricted attention that is part of the struggle with anxiety. If we're always turning away from our emotions, it can be difficult to identify and understand them. If we're using all of our mental energy to push thoughts and images away, it can be difficult to focus on what is happening in the moment.

Solution 2: Mindfulness Helps Us Stop Rigidly and Automatically Avoiding Our Experience

Let's return for a moment to our souring relationship with the troublesome employee, Chet. Imagine that, before firing Chet, you decide to speak to Wilma in human resources about your problem. Wilma suggests that the three of you meet regularly for the next few weeks in an attempt to repair the relationship. Maybe you're skeptical; after all, you've been trying to fix this relationship for a long time to no avail. But, you decide, why not give this relationship one last chance?

One of the first things Wilma does is pass along Chet's employee file. As you read through the documents, you're surprised to learn the ways in which Chet is actually quite helpful to the company. Perhaps you still don't love having him around, but you acknowledge that he contributes something valuable and unique to the workplace. As you get to know Chet better, you start to understand his idiosyncrasies and accept them as a part of who he is.

At Wilma's urging you also try a new technique to deal with Chet when he makes a mistake. Rather than responding with harsh criticism, which you had hoped would

> *Mindfulness helps us experience even uncomfortable emotions long enough to learn what they're really telling us to do.*

be motivating (after all, isn't threatening to fire someone the best way to motivate him?), Wilma suggests that you first try to understand what happened and then encourage Chet to try something different next time. Maybe Chet was misinformed during his training, or perhaps he's just having a rough day. This new understanding of your employee allows you to feel compassionate toward him while also encouraging him to improve his performance. You take a leap of faith and try this new compassionate but firm approach. You are pleased and surprised to see his performance improve steadily.

Think of what just changed in your relationship with Chet as what could change in your relationship with anxiety—and any other emotion you're usually tempted to avoid—when you turn toward your experience and take a fresh look at a familiar response. You observed Chet with gentle curiosity and found out some surprising facts about him, just as you could about the anxiety you've come to abhor. You extended compassion to him and his human foibles, just as you could to yourself and your natural, instinctive fear responses.

As a result, you've changed your relationship with Chet, and now you'll no longer feel compelled to avoid him at all costs. You don't have to become his best friend or wander around the halls searching for him. But if you're in the break room and Chet shows up, you can just slide over, make room for him, and keep going about your business.

Similarly, because mindfulness changes the relationship you have with anxiety and the rest of your internal experience, it also reduces your urge to avoid. If you begin to see the value of anxiety and other emotions, bring compassion and understanding to your experience, and come to recognize that you are not defined or controlled by your anxiety, you may no longer see your reactions as dangerous and threatening. You probably will never actively seek out painful thoughts or negative emotions, just for the heck of it. But if engaging in your life in a meaningful way means that pain might show up every once in a while, mindfulness helps you slide over to make room.

Problem 3: Struggles with Anxiety Pull Us Away from What Matters Most

Being engaged in a constant battle against your internal experiences and trying to avoid anxiety-related thoughts, feelings, and emotions is time intensive and exhausting. As a result, when we're in the thick of this struggle, activities such as connecting with friends and family, cultivating new relationships, pursuing career challenges, nurturing our talents and interests, exploring our spirituality, and participating in our community are placed on the back burner. "As soon as we win this battle," we promise ourselves, "we will get back to the business of living."

> *Rejecting all fear and anxiety may mean narrowing your life in ways you never intended.*

At first glance, this plan seems reasonable. Why not invest all your time and effort into conquering your anxiety problems once and for all and then freely pursue the things in life that matter most to you? This problem-solving strategy works for other kinds of problems. For example, it makes sense to hold off on watching television until you finish writing a report that is due the next day. It would be reasonable to put off going out for a walk until you finish loading the dishwasher.

The problem with applying this approach to managing your anxiety is that experiencing fear and anxiety, vulnerable and irrational thoughts, and uncomfortable physical sensations is an inherent part of being human. No amount of self-determination, motivation, discipline, therapy, or medication will help us overcome our humanness. So essentially if we take this approach we get stuck putting our life on hold while pursuing an unattainable goal.

Even if by chance we've been lucky enough to hold on to a few of the things that matter most to us, our anxiety and worry may make it difficult to freely enjoy and appreciate them. Struggling with anxiety can make everything feel like a chore, like we're going through the motions but missing out on the rewards. Being locked in a struggle with anxiety can make all of us feel like spectators in our own lives.

Solution 3: Mindfulness Promotes Engagement and Participation

Mindfulness not only helps us become aware of the obvious and subtle ways in which our attempts to avoid anxiety have set restrictions on the way we live our lives; it also allows us to honestly evaluate the life directions that are most personally meaningful and valuable to our sense of vitality and fulfillment. Learning how to take a mindful stance toward painful thoughts and feelings decreases their intensity and inhibitive power, freeing us up to pursue valued life directions.

> *Mindfulness can show you how much you've given up to avoid anxiety and what it is you most want back in your life.*

Mindfulness increases our willingness to experience the full range of thoughts, emotions, and sensations that arise when we are fully engaged and participating in life.

When Keisha (from the beginning of this chapter) began to practice mindfulness, she became aware of how focusing on her anxiety was pulling her away from connections with people she cared about. Keisha always knew that she valued relationships; in fact, her drive to perform perfectly in social situations was driven by the desire to be loved and accepted by others. Keisha assumed that exuding confidence was the best way to secure friends and that fixing her internal "flaws" was the only way she could become acceptable to others. Given her firm belief in the potential usefulness of this strategy, Keisha was reluctant to bring beginner's mind (a mindfulness skill introduced in Chapter 5) to more closely examining her behavior, but she was soon startled by the reality that the more she focused on "fixing" herself the less she actually connected with others. Mindfulness helped Keisha become more aware of her own behavior and its unintended consequences. Also, mindfulness practice helped Keisha notice in the moment when her old self-ruminative habits kicked in. At these times, although her attention was drawn toward self-focus, Keisha learned to purposefully expand her awareness and began to notice subtle cues that others were trying to send her, like when Joslin was seeking her reassurance and Andres was expressing interest. Keisha also became more in tune with the full range of her responses in social situations. Although she felt fear and apprehension sitting with classmates before a presentation, she also noticed feelings of self-compassion, camaraderie, and pride. Keisha's increased awareness helped her recognize how important these moments of connection were to her, so that she was able to choose to respond to her friends, rather than pulling into herself due to her anxiety. Her attention to these relationships helped to reduce her sense of unease and loneliness and led her to feel significantly more satisfied with her life.

Embarking on a New Path

Our goal is to introduce you to the concept of mindfulness and provide you with practices aimed at helping you change the relationship you have with anxiety and related emotions, thoughts, and physical sensations. You may have already noticed this relationship changing a bit as you learned about the nature of your responses and began to pay attention to them. But don't worry if you haven't. Mindfulness is a skill that becomes more automatic and natural with patience and faithful practice. In the next chapter we start teaching you a wide range of practices so that you can gradually develop this new type of awareness.

In the next chapter, we start by having you notice different physical sensations like breathing, tensing your muscles, and relaxing. We also ask you to pay attention to your environment in a more careful and curious way—noticing what it is like to eat, being aware of sounds, realizing when you first become anxious. The discoveries that our clients (and others) make with these preliminary exercises make it easier to approach the more challenging mindfulness practices such as bringing curiosity and compassion to anxiety and other painful thoughts and emotions.

As you work on increasing your mindfulness, in the following chapters, we tell you what the most up-to-date psychological research says about how emotions function to enhance our lives and how attempts to control them only increase our struggle. Meanwhile, we encourage you to explore what matters most to you, to examine how anxiety and avoidance prevent you from living life to the fullest, and to develop a plan to work through obstacles to valued living.

Our experience has been that the more time and effort you can devote to this program, the more you will reap its benefits. Many people who struggle with anxiety have extremely busy lives. If trying to pile one more thing onto your already heavy load seems daunting, remember that struggling with anxiety is a habit that takes some time to develop. Developing new habits to take the place of the struggle will naturally take some time and practice. So we suggest you set aside some time to read, complete the exercises, and engage in mindfulness practice. Very quickly, you'll find that you've begun integrating these new techniques and skills into your daily life.

As suggested at the beginning of the book, we hope you take an open and curious stance and try the exercises even if they seem unfamiliar or outright awkward. Give each exercise a try, even if you don't think it will help. Then use your newly developed observation skills and your own fresh experience to determine which strategies or methods are most useful to you.

Regardless of how much you are currently struggling with anxiety or how long you have lived with your anxiety symptoms, keep in mind that you already possess all you need to live a valued, satisfying, and meaningful life. We hope you can use the strategies and methods described throughout the book, developed through our research and clinical work in the areas of anxiety and mindfulness, to change your relationship with anxiety and embark on a new path.

EXERCISE **Paying closer attention to fear and anxiety in a new way**

In Chapter 1 we suggested that you begin observing your response when you notice yourself beginning to feel anxious or afraid. If you have been trying this, you have been practicing an early form of mindfulness! If not, you can begin doing so now. The idea is to carry a small notebook and record your anxious responses in the moment when you notice them, at least once or twice a day. In Chapter 1, we suggested recording the day, situation, and any anxious responses. A new challenge is to break down your anxious response into components. So, when you notice anxiety arising, take a moment and separately note your thoughts, emotions, physical sensations, and behaviors. It can be really helpful to explore each domain to see whether you notice the subtle nuances in your responding. Remember, this method of observation involves *turning toward something that we would usually avoid* and *taking a fresh look at a familiar response*. In addition, when you notice critical thoughts about your responses arising, try to bring *kindness and compassion* to your responses. Remember what you've learned already about how natural it is to be anxious and how these are habitual responses that you've learned over time, not signs of weakness or flaws. We will work together to develop this self-compassion throughout the rest of the book, so don't be frustrated if you find it challenging to bring compassion right away. Just try it out for now and see what you notice.

4

an introduction to mindfulness

NOTICING A SKILL YOU ALREADY POSSESS

One somewhat snowy Monday morning, the elementary school my (S. M. O.) son Sam goes to was closed due to the weather. Unfortunately, the university where I teach was still open, and I had to teach a class that morning. My husband and I decided it would make the most sense for Sam to go to work with me. My son usually enjoys "helping me teach," and we could return home as soon as my office hours ended. I raced around a bit, pulling my stuff together, and off we went to the train station.

Sam settled into a seat next to the window on the train bound to Boston. I told him I needed to prepare my lecture and asked him to read his book or sit quietly and look out the window while I worked. I slung my backpack onto the empty seat next to me, pulled out my book, laptop, cereal bar, and water bottle, stuck my ticket in the slot to be punched, and settled into my morning routine. As the train moved along, I glanced through the chapters I had assigned for the day's class and made lecture notes on my computer while gobbling down my breakfast. When we pulled into the next station, I grudgingly moved my bag and scooted over next to Sam to make room for another passenger without missing a keystroke. Sam kept up a steady monologue, describing the iced-over lake we passed, the yachts covered with tarps for the winter, and finally the hulking machinery at a nearby construction site. As I put the finishing touches on my lecture, I noticed he was on his knees, peering out the window, and sternly reminded him to stay seated. Moments later we pulled into the station, our trip successful. I had finished my breakfast, prepared for class, and kept my son entertained and reasonably well behaved.

But consider for a moment how, with a few small changes, my experience might have been different. Imagine, for instance, that I had focused my attention on the cereal bar while I ate ... noticing the many different textures and flavors all merged together: crunchy oats, raisins bursting with juice, the earthy flavor of almonds ... noticing how each bite gave me sustenance and energy for the day ... observing how the water I drank quenched my thirst.

Now imagine that I had brought my full attention to my work. I might more fully feel the satisfaction of creating a lesson plan that could spark a lively class discussion.

Imagine the small but meaningful interactions I could have had that morning. What if I had made eye contact with the conductor as she punched my ticket and caught the grateful nod she sent my way for having my ticket ready and making her morning work just a little easier? What if I had noticed that older gentleman seated beside me who looked a bit nervous about riding into Boston? Maybe if I had acknowledged him, he would have asked me his questions about how to transfer from the commuter rail to the subway. Helping him out and seeing his relief might have brought me a moment of pleasure.

What if I had turned my full attention to Sam and saw the wonder and excitement in his eyes as he took in all the details of the train ride? What if I saw beyond what I know my son to be—an energetic 10-year-old with a love of sports and video games—and noticed his moment-to-moment reactions to the trip? Imagine the love, pride, and compassion I might have felt.

Multitasking and Automatic Pilot: Thriving or Surviving in the 21st Century?

On the surface, these two commutes do not really seem radically different. Multitasking on the train is a ritual for many commuters. There is no real harm in living this way. Or is there? And how much benefit can one really get from observing the moment as it unfolds? With all the problems we face, how could such a small thing make any difference at all? And most important, what does all of this have to do with anxiety? We begin to explore these questions in this chapter and continue to consider them throughout the rest of the book.

Multitasking has become part of our everyday lives. The teenager planted on the couch in front of the television, typing his homework assignment onto the laptop perched on his knees, shoveling down a snack, and instant messaging (IMing) with his friend about the new girl in their chemistry class. The mother holding her fussy baby in one arm while stirring the pot of sauce on the stove, helping a coworker problem-solve a customer service issue over the phone, and stealing an occasional glance at the television.

Sometimes we multitask in a somewhat more subtle way, engaging in one activity while thinking about another. Remember Eric (introduced in Chapter 2), who couldn't seem to enjoy quality time alone with his daughter because he was preoccupied with work worries and couldn't focus at work because he was preoccupied with worries about losing his cherished family? We may try to engage in one valued action while at the same time worrying about another. Sometimes this process occurs outside of our control. But other times it reflects our attempts to manage multiple demands. Picture a father paused by his daughter's bedroom door, trying to nod sympathetically as his teenager complains about school, all the while distracted by worries about missing the train and being late for work. Think of a woman on a much-needed "dinner date" who tries to appear attentive to her partner while ruminating over the sharp criticism she received from her boss earlier in the day.

> *Even if you're* doing *only one thing, you could be multitasking by* worrying *about another at the same time.*

When our attention is stretched thin by multitasking, we begin to operate on autopilot in some domains. The teen juggling four activities from the couch may get engrossed in the TV program that just came on, but when it's over he probably won't be able to tell you exactly what his snack consisted of or how it tasted. The mother on the phone may momentarily tune out her coworker while trying to recall the exact location of the oregano in the pantry. The ability to simultaneously execute multiple actions without giving each behavior significant thought can be useful. When you first learn to drive a stick shift, your attention is pretty much consumed with coordinating the clutch and the gas pedal, making it difficult to navigate through an unfamiliar neighborhood. But a veteran driver expends very little cognitive energy on shifting gears and can easily watch for street signs or casually chat with a passenger while doing so.

Multitasking is considered by some to be a necessary evil. After all, given the multiple demands of modern living, how else will we succeed in our busy lives? The reality is multitasking has some significant downsides. What may work for driving does not always work for other domains of living. Multitasking on a regular basis, particularly in an automatic, habitual way, increases stress and decreases productivity. There is a limited amount of information we can pay attention to and remember, particularly when we are overloaded with stimuli. We might be able to solve a crossword puzzle with soft classical music playing in the background. But research shows that multitasking is inefficient, and those who engage in multitasking actually perform worse on cognitive and memory tasks. Although we may be able to engage and disengage the clutch effortlessly while taking in the traffic conditions, texting, putting on make-up, or talking on a cell phone while driving can result in tragedy. There are also social and personal costs to multitasking. The coworker on the phone with the busy mother may feel frustrated that she is not getting clear advice. The daughter may feel that her father doesn't care or take her problems seriously. The diner will likely not feel nurtured or sustained by her night out with her partner. Although we may try valiantly to meet multiple competing demands, the end result of multitasking often is not entirely satisfying.

In addition to interfering with our concentration and productivity and diminishing our connections with others, moving through life on autopilot can prevent us from making significant life changes. Consider Luana, who has struggled with social anxiety all her life. Luana just started a new job and hopes to build relationships with her coworkers. Although she constantly fears that people are scrutinizing and evaluating her, she is also yearning for a deeper connection with others. Luana is single, with few friends, and she is lonely.

For 2 weeks leading up to her start date, Luana imagined what it would be like to socialize with her coworkers. She imagined going out for drinks after work, maybe even seeing a movie on the weekend with a group of friends from work. For her first few days on the job, Luana

The Obvious and Hidden Costs of Multitasking

ATTENTION AND MEMORY PROBLEMS

- Your school or job performance may suffer.
- Managing household chores can be difficult.
- You may fail to pick up subtle, nonverbal messages from those around you.
- You may not adequately learn from your experiences because your ability to perceive the consequences of moment-to-moment actions is limited.

STRAINED RELATIONSHIPS

- The important people in your life may feel neglected even though you believe you're spending sufficient time with them.
- You may inadvertently send signals that you're not interested and don't care about those around you.
- Your inability to pick up subtle, nonverbal messages from people you care about may lead to hurt feelings and misunderstandings.

DISSATISFACTION AND DISCONTENT IN YOUR WORK, RELATIONSHIPS, AND HOBBIES

- It can seem like you are just going through the motions.
- You may feel like a spectator in your own life.
- You may fail to notice and fully experience the enjoyable aspects of your relationships, work, or leisure activities.
- What you're trying to avoid can become more important than what you want to achieve.

CONFUSION AND HOPELESSNESS

- You might feel as if you're working extremely hard to balance competing demands, yet your efforts don't seem to pay off.
- You may feel at a loss as to how you can improve your situation.

was filled with both anticipation and anxiety. What if everyone thought she was too old or boring to hang out with? If someone approached her and engaged in small talk, would she be able to think of ways to keep the conversation going? Then one day, while she was focused on trying to understand a complex spreadsheet open on her desktop, Luana was startled by the appearance of two women from the sales department leaning into her doorway. "Join us for a quick lunch around the corner?" the younger of the two casually requested. Before she was even aware of her action, Luana heard herself begging off. "No thanks," she stammered. "I usually bring my own and work straight through lunch." In a matter of seconds Luana's fear had spiked, her habitual avoidance response kicked in, and she felt an immediate sense of relief followed by a wave of sorrow. Although Luana values social connections, her desire to avoid uncomfortable situations makes it very difficult for her to be willing to experience fear and anxiety.

This sort of thing happens all the time. We want to do something that is important to us, but we don't want to feel uncomfortable. So we choose to avoid. And the relief we feel is so reinforcing that it just strengthens the habit. A cycle is formed, usually outside the realm of our typical awareness, where fear leads to avoidance, which leads to more avoidance.

If we pay close attention to our thoughts, emotions, and urges to avoid, there is some hope of breaking that cycle. Remember, emotions do not cause behaviors; they just bring on a strong urge to behave in a certain way. If we can catch this urge before we act, more choices become available to us. But if we're not paying close attention, the habit of avoidance can kick in. Living on automatic pilot means our lives may be shaped more by what we are avoiding than what we are pursuing.

Mindfulness: A Way to Step Back into Your Life

The difference between the two commutes described at the beginning of the chapter is that during the second trip I was practicing mindfulness. *Mindfulness* is a term that brings up different images and meanings for different people. You may associate it with the spiritual traditions of Buddhism. Or you may think of it as a pop-culture, new-age fad. You may have heard about the health benefits of mindfulness and be intrigued and interested in learning more. Or you may not have a clear sense of what it is at all. See the sidebar on pages 82–83.

Put simply, mindfulness is a specific way of paying attention to things. It involves **purposefully expanding your attention** to take in both what you are experiencing inside—your thoughts, feelings, and physical sensations—and what is happening around you. But the kind of attention you bring to noticing is an essential aspect of this practice. Mindfulness involves **bringing a gentle and honest curiosity** to your experiences. It involves looking at familiar thoughts, people, and situations with a **fresh perspective**, as if you had never encountered them before.

> *Paying close attention to an urge to avoid discomfort can help us break the cycle of fear → avoidance → relief → restricted life.*

One of the most challenging mindfulness skills is **self-compassion.** Typically, we label and judge the stream of experiences we have without even giving the process much thought. Sitting in my office, I hear a variety of sounds that I quickly categorize: "blaring horn"—annoying; "ambulance siren"—danger; "laughing coworker"—fun. I react the same way to a stream of internal experiences: the thought "I need to go to the dry cleaner"—distracting; the feeling of sadness—bad, to be avoided; a sensation of tension—frustration. Mindfulness involves understanding that making snap judgments is an adaptive part of human nature. After all, it is in my best interest to quickly judge the sour taste of milk as disgusting and to judge things I fear as threatening and dangerous. And mindfulness involves being able to accept, and even welcome, what can't be changed, rather than struggling to control things beyond our control.

> *Self-compassion can help us turn the corner from rejecting discomfort to accepting our experience, even if only for a moment longer than usual.*

So, learning to be compassionate toward our own responses means that when we notice thoughts, sensations, or emotions, we try to be gentle with ourselves, remembering that these responses are natural and an inherent part of being human, rather than criticizing ourselves for having them. And when we inevitably do have critical reactions to fear, doubt, and other internal experiences (as these are overlearned habits and part of being human), we can be gentle and compassionate with ourselves

Common Questions and Concerns about Mindfulness

Isn't mindfulness part of Buddhism? What if I have different spiritual or religious beliefs?

The term *mindfulness* comes from Buddhism, but psychology has begun to recognize that mindfulness (removed from the religious context) may be used to improve physical and emotional well-being. Although many of the ideas we suggest here are consistent with Eastern philosophies and traditions, we do not focus on the religious parts of mindfulness, and we believe this approach can be useful no matter what your religious or spiritual preference. In fact, mindful awareness is a part of religious practices in many traditions and can also be practiced without any religious connection.

Isn't mindfulness just some sort of new-age fad?

Although mindfulness has become part of our popular culture, the suggestions we make throughout this book are based on more than 10 years of research that has been conducted by us and many other scientists.

I don't have the time to practice mindfulness.

There is debate in the field as to how much mindfulness practice is needed to experience benefits in health and well-being. Our research and the research of others suggests that more practice is associated with greater benefit. However, after completing an intensive mindfulness training program, some people find that a practice as simple and brief as focusing on their breath during the day helps them maintain gains. In our experience, the time we spend practicing mindfulness is well spent because it helps us do other tasks more efficiently and with more satisfaction.

I don't have the right personality to practice mindfulness.

We have never worked with an anxious person who felt comfortable with the idea of just sitting and noticing. Yet our clients find that, with practice, they can develop a mindfulness practice, just like building any new habit. If you struggle with anxiety and stress, it should feel strange and unfamiliar to practice breathing and other formal mindfulness exercises. If we offered you a technique that was similar to the ones you have been using to cope already (unsuccessfully), it would probably not be helpful.

I did a little mindfulness in my yoga class. Is this anything different?

Yes and no. Practicing meditation or yoga is definitely consistent with the type of mindfulness practice we describe here. But we bring our expertise as psychologists who study anxiety to consider how mindfulness can be used to reduce self-criticism, to decrease the intensity of negative mood states, and to increase life satisfaction.

Is mindfulness the same as relaxation?

Again, the answer is yes and no. Although mindfulness practice sometimes produces a state that quiets the mind and brings on feelings of calmness, that is not always the case. Mindfulness is used to bring you into contact with the present moment. If the present moment is distressing, mindfulness will not eliminate that distress. But mindfulness may allow you to experience the distress differently and to participate in your life while you are feeling distress.

for *that* response as well. As we explore in more depth in the following chapters, this continual practice of self-compassion will help us break the cycle of reactivity and criticism that often drives our anxiety and break our habit of avoiding discomfort so that we are free to engage more fully in our lives.

Mindfulness Defined

1. Noticing
   - Becoming fully aware of the thoughts, feelings, physical sensations, and images that you experience
   - Observing all the details of your environment

2. Bringing curiosity and interest to new as well as familiar experiences
   - Approaching experiences with openness
   - Viewing events "as they are" instead of "as what you know" or "as you wish they were" or "as you fear they are"

3. Practicing self-compassion
   - Noticing the pull to label, judge, and react to experiences
   - Acknowledging that the reactions we have are part of being human
   - Accepting what cannot be controlled
   - Treating yourself (and ultimately others) with kindness and care
   - Treating your experiences with kindness and care

Before we talk about mindfulness any further, we would like you to do a quick breathing exercise. It takes only a few minutes, but to really get the most out of this chapter it is important to do this exercise before you read on (even if you have tried mindfulness before). Find a quiet, comfortable spot where you can sit for 5 minutes and not be disturbed. Bring a pad of paper and something to write with so that you can jot down anything you notice about the experience or any reactions you have. Make sure to set a timer on your watch or cell phone so that you know when 5 minutes is up. Read the instructions below and then put the book aside to practice.

Ways to Sit for Mindfulness Practice

Bringing awareness to the way you are sitting prior to starting your practice will help you to practice mindfulness without being needlessly distracted by physical sensations of discomfort (although sensations will still arise as part of your practice).

SITTING ON THE FLOOR

- *With legs folded.* One option is to sit on the floor with your legs folded in front of you. Use one or two cushions so that your buttocks are elevated. Place your legs folded, in front of you on the floor, one in front of the other. Your weight should be balanced evenly across your buttocks and your two knees, with your buttocks elevated above your legs. This puts much less strain on your knees than having your buttocks and knees on an even plane. Straighten your spine and drop your shoulders so that you are in a comfortable upright position. You can place your hands on your thighs or bring your fingertips together in your lap, whichever feels more comfortable.

- *In a supported kneeling position.* Another option is to kneel with a cushion lifting your buttocks off the ground. If you are using a traditional meditation cushion, you may find it helpful to turn the cushion on its edge and place it between your thighs, sitting on the top edge of the cushion. Rest your hands, palms down, in a comfortable position on your thighs so that you are neither pulled forward nor arched back. Again, straighten your spine so that you are sitting evenly and alertly.

SITTING IN A CHAIR

Another option is to sit in a straight-backed chair. Rest both feet on the floor in front of you. Straighten your spine and sit upright, rather than leaning against the back of the chair. Place your hands, palms down, on your thighs so that your shoulders are relaxed.

POSTURE

As you begin practicing, be sure to bring awareness to your posture. All of us tend to slouch our shoulders or bend our lower back. Both will cause discomfort and make practice more challenging. If you notice any soreness after you practice, bring attention to that part of your body the next time you sit and be sure you choose a position that does not put unnecessary strain on that part of your body. It can be helpful to imagine that a string is pulling your head upward so that you can find a lifted, straight spine when you begin sitting. Remember that a straight spine will still have a curve in your lumbar, so don't try to straighten that out. Over time this position will become a habit, so you won't have to think about it as much.

The Mindfulness of Breath Exercise

1. Close your eyes or allow your gaze to rest softly on a spot on the floor in front of you.

2. Notice where you feel the breath in your body and allow your attention to rest in this spot. It may be in your belly, the back of your throat, or your nostrils.

3. Keep your focus on your breath, "being with" each in breath for its full duration and with each out breath for its full duration. Imagine you are riding the waves of your own breathing.

4. Each time you notice that your mind has wandered off the breath, gently bring your attention back to the place you feel your breath and the feeling of each in breath and out breath.

5. Each time your mind wanders, all you need to do is gently bring it back to your breath, again and again and again.

6. If you notice thoughts that you aren't doing this right or you aren't good at it, just notice them and again gently bring your attention back to your breath, again and again. These are just thoughts; they don't mean you aren't doing it right.

Congratulations! If you have never tried mindfulness before, you have just completed your first practice. Let's review what was simple or easy about this exercise. It wasn't very time consuming (even the busiest among us can usually find 5 minutes). The exercise doesn't require any specialized equipment. It involves something that you already do on a regular basis—breathing. You had only one task, which was to pay attention to your breath. And finally, there is nothing mysterious about doing it.

Although this exercise is amazingly simple, we are sure you noticed that it also can be quite challenging. Each of us has our own unique experience when we practice mindfulness, but some reactions are pretty common. Following is a list of things that some people notice when they do this exercise. Notice which of the statements describe your personal experience and acknowledge any other reactions you had that are not listed.

Common Reactions to the Breathing Exercise

- "I wasn't sure I was breathing the right way."
- "I started taking really shallow breaths."
- "I felt short of breath."
- "I felt self-conscious about my breathing."
- "Five minutes seemed to last forever."
- "I kept opening my eyes to check the time."
- "I felt restless and fidgety."
- "I couldn't keep my mind on the task."
- "I kept thinking about things I need to get done."
- "I had the thought 'This is a waste of time.'"
- "I had the thought 'How will this help me?'"
- "I had the thought 'I can't do this right.'"
- "I felt anxious and uncomfortable."
- "I had the thought 'I believe mindfulness might be helpful for many people, but not me.'"

The Lessons We Learn from Mindfulness

Most people find paying attention to their breath for 5 minutes extremely challenging. This is why we asked you to try it before reading on. Until you actually try to keep your attention on your breath for 5 minutes, it can seem like a very simple task.

When people first try mindfulness, they typically make a judgment as to whether they were "successful." Did you have any thoughts like that? Even though we don't know anything about you or the unique experience you just had, we can confidently conclude that you succeeded. How can that be? Because there is absolutely no way to fail during mindfulness practice. Certainly one benefit of the breathing exercise (and mindfulness practice in general) is that, over time, you may develop the ability to notice more easily when your attention has strayed and to guide it more easily toward some target (e.g., your breath, the meal you are eating, the conversation you are in). This part of mindfulness definitely improves with practice. But it's important to understand that mindfulness is a process. No one ever achieves a total and final state of mindfulness. It is a way of being in one moment that comes and goes. In fact, it is often said that mindfulness is losing our focus 100 times and returning to it 101 times.

Beginners often judge themselves negatively if they can't keep their attention on their breathing for 5 minutes (or even 5 seconds). But an extremely important second benefit of mindfulness practice is simply noticing what happens when we try to bring our attention to our breath. There are many lessons to be learned about how our mind works and how it affects our behavior if we pay close attention.

We go through our daily lives thinking all kinds of thoughts. Our minds are very busy, and they often hop from topic to topic. But rarely do we actually notice our thinking or watch our thoughts as they race through our mind. In other words, we might think, "I have absolutely no patience," but we don't usually think, "I am observing that I am having the thought that I have no patience." We think, "I am anxious," not, "I am experiencing a feeling of anxiety." We typically operate in a state of being fused with our thoughts, emotions, or physical sensations. When we are mindful, we get the chance to step back, at least for a moment, and observe them.

Although it is common to have mundane thoughts during mindfulness practice, like, "I wonder what I should have for lunch," or, "I need to stop at the store on my way home," most people also have self-critical thoughts like the ones in the box on page 87. If the average person has this reaction to watching the breath, imagine the kinds of thoughts that are common when we take risks or allow ourselves to feel vulnerable.

Observing our thoughts instead of just thinking them gives us a moment to choose to act on them differently.

Where do all these judgmental thoughts come from? First, they are part of our culture. We often get the message that being critical or "hard" on ourselves is desirable and motivating. Mira thinks she can reach her weight-loss goals by harshly judging herself as lazy and weak. Gabe is disgusted by his fear of public speaking and tries to be "tough" on himself in an effort to conquer his fear. Although this approach is not helping them, they both think that if they were to "let up" things would only get worse. There is little evidence that self-criticism motivates lasting, positive changes, but many people continue to live by that rule. We also collect critical, judgmental thoughts through our own personal experiences. Interactions with family, teachers, friends, bosses, coworkers, and partners can teach us that it's wrong to feel a certain emotion, have a certain thought, or behave in a particular way.

Important Lessons to Be Learned from Mindfulness

- Our minds are very busy.
- Although we can notice our thoughts (emotions, physical sensations), we usually just have them.
- We are often "fused" with our internal experiences.
- Our thoughts are often harsh and critical.

How Can Mindfulness Help If You Are Anxious?

People who struggle with stress or anxiety often think that mindfulness is a technique that can be used to calm or relax them. Mindfulness of the breath or other exercises sometimes do quiet the mind and bring momentary peace. But mindfulness is much more than that. As you will learn from this book, mindfulness can help you better understand yourself and make the kind of lasting life changes that bring satisfaction and fulfillment. It can help you break unproductive habits and open up choices for you. But it does require you to become aware of, and open up to, all of your experiences, even the difficult ones.

At this point you might be thinking, "Gee, thanks, but I'm already painfully aware of the negative, judgmental thoughts I have about myself—especially when I'm under stress!" In fact, you may be wondering whether you should have spent the price of this book on something more soothing, like a ticket to a nice little romantic comedy. After all, you bought this book hoping it would help you become *less* aware of those thoughts, not *more*. Please bear with us. We're confident that you'll see that mindfully experiencing painful thoughts is very different from the way most of us typically operate.

Let's imagine what is going on in Natalie's head when she gets really stressed and nervous. Natalie works as a middle school teacher in a small suburban town. Late one Friday afternoon, as she is packing up to leave for the day, she receives a call from the principal. Mr. Freedman tells her that a parent of one of her pupils has called to complain that Natalie is disorganized in assigning and managing homework assignments. The principal asks Natalie to come to his office so that they can discuss the situation. Mr. Freedman wants to hear about Natalie's homework policy, her perspective on why the student and her parent might be upset, and how she might want to address the complaint. Natalie feels a surge of panic. She quickly hangs up the phone, bolts out of the classroom, and heads down the hall.

On the way, Natalie is engrossed in an inner monologue. "Oh no, I can't believe this is happening to me. I can't stand that student. And you have got to love these parents. They give their kids everything they want, let them watch television and play video games all the time, and don't get involved in their education one bit, until they have some complaint. Ugh. I shouldn't have changed the homework assignment at the last minute. Why didn't I just stick to the regular social studies curriculum? What an idiot I was to think that a current-events assignment was a fun and creative addition. A veteran teacher wouldn't have made that mistake. Or she would have planned the assignment further in advance. Why didn't the student or the parent just contact me directly? Do I seem unapproachable? Mr. Freedman must think I can't manage my own classroom. This is the last thing he wants to deal with on a Friday. What should I do? I am so stressed out I can't even think straight."

Natalie takes a seat across the desk from the principal, the tension apparent in her stiff shoulders and trembling hands. "That student has always been a problem in my classroom," she begins, her voice building in volume. "He never does his homework on time, and his notebook is always a mess. The parent is unhappy that I gave her precious son a C on his last report card, and this is her way of retaliating. Kids today don't think they need to earn a grade; they believe they deserve an A just for showing up to class. Where was his mother when he failed the last quiz?

She certainly didn't help him study or contact me to develop a plan for him to improve his performance."

Although Mr. Freedman tries to express his perspective on the situation, Natalie is too distracted by her own thoughts to pay attention to what he's saying. She feels as if she's being attacked. "I just need to get out of here and relax" is all she can think. Plus, she already knows from experience exactly what Mr. Freedman's response will be. He always wants teachers to stick to the curriculum, and the parents are always right in his eyes. Somewhat abruptly, Natalie ends the discussion by agreeing to call the parent and arrange a meeting to discuss the issue. However, when she gets back to her classroom, she feels like she is way too emotional to deal with the situation and decides to leave. On her way out, Natalie calls to the principal, "No one was home, I left a message," and she immediately feels better as she slips into her car and pulls out of the parking lot, leaving the mess behind.

Unfortunately, that night Natalie can't sleep. She keeps replaying the scenario in her mind, and she feels extremely tense and irritable. Finally, she gets up, takes two sleeping pills, and turns on the television, hoping it will lull her to sleep. But her thoughts keep replaying the scene at the school, and she is dreading having to deal with the situation on Monday.

In this situation Natalie clearly had some awareness of her painful thoughts and feelings. Yet she was definitely not bringing mindfulness to the situation. Let's imagine how this scenario could have unfolded differently.

When Natalie receives the call from her principal, she tells Mr. Freedman she will come down to his office in just a few moments. She feels strong emotions arising and notices her thoughts racing, so Natalie decides to take a few moments to bring her attention to her inner experience. "I am definitely experiencing anger at the student and the parent for complaining to the principal instead of contacting me directly. But I also notice some feelings of sadness, embarrassment, and fear. Of course, I am having the thought that this means I am a terrible teacher and that Mr. Freedman is angry with or disappointed in me. I'm sure that's a reaction any teacher would have in this situation. I'm also having some thoughts that the student is irresponsible and the parent extremely difficult. No surprise—this is definitely a pattern I recognize. When I feel vulnerable or threatened, my mind generates all these thoughts blaming others to protect me from pain. When I'm pumped up with anger, it makes me feel strong—well, at least in the moment. I also know from experience that acting on that anger, without carefully considering all of my options and choosing the action that is most consistent with the kind of teacher and employee I want to be, often backfires."

Natalie's thoughts began to race: "Ugh. I shouldn't have changed the homework assignment at the last minute. Why didn't I just stick to the regular social studies curriculum? What an idiot I was to think that adding a current-events assignment was going to seem fun and creative. A veteran teacher wouldn't have made that mistake." For a moment, Natalie is tangled up in these thoughts. She is fused with her thinking, feeling, and judging and not observing the process. Then she notices what's happening and brings her attention back to an observer perspective. "Almost got swept up in that familiar script," she acknowledges.

Natalie purposefully pays keen attention to both her internal experience and Mr. Freedman as she sits across the desk from the principal. She has the thought "I know he will take the parent's side," but rather than getting caught up in her thoughts, she brings her attention back to what Mr. Freedman is actually saying. Natalie notices the lines of concern on Mr. Freedman's face as he speaks. She hears the genuineness in his voice as he discusses his perspective, wondering whether there is a way to turn this into an opportunity to engage the parent in her son's education. Natalie notices that the intensity of her emotions began to subside as they discuss possible options for dealing with the problem. Her first thought is to ask Mr. Freedman to deal with the irate parent. But she realizes that to be the kind of teacher she wants to be, she will have to talk to the parent directly.

Natalie heads back to the classroom to make the call. She notices a surge of fear and the thought "I am feeling too emotional to deal with this situation right now." Natalie also notices a strong urge to leave the problem behind and deal with it after the weekend. But she recognizes this as an old pattern: avoid a difficult situation to reduce her discomfort. Natalie takes a moment simply to observe these thoughts, feelings, and urges without judging them or acting on them. She notices that they grow and peak and then subside just a little bit. She is clearly still experiencing painful thoughts and emotions, but she chooses to place the call. It is a difficult interaction with the parent, but she leaves the building satisfied that she has done the best she can in the situation.

Taking the First Step

The example of Natalie demonstrates how mindfulness can help us notice what we are experiencing, make choices about how we want to respond, and increase our willingness to allow difficult thoughts and feelings without struggling to get rid of them. Throughout the rest of the book we take you little by little toward moving through your anxiety to engage in your life. The first step in this process is developing a daily mindfulness practice. If you're anything like us, your first reaction might be "Hold on, I don't have time to add another thing to my full plate." The good news is that mindfulness can be integrated very easily into a busy life.

EXERCISE **Investing in yourself with mindfulness practice**

We recommend that you invest 5 minutes a day for the next week into your own self-care. Specifically, we would like you to consider doing the mindfulness of breath exercise for at least 5 minutes each day for the next week.

Notice your thoughts, feelings, and physical sensations during the exercise so that you can jot them down later. See if you can bring a lighthearted curiosity to the experience. The goal is not to see how long you can focus on your breath or to calm all your fears and worries. Instead, take these 5 minutes to become better acquainted with what happens when you slow down and breathe. Get to know how your mind works and where it likes to wander. Practice acknowledging its frenetic pace and its tendency to worry and criticize. Then guide your attention back to your breath like you might lead a reluctant toddler away from the playground and toward home for a much-needed rest.

Things to Keep in Mind When Practicing Mindfulness

1. Practice becoming fully aware of your internal reactions and the world around you.
2. Notice when your attention narrows; allow it to expand.
3. Practice patience with the present moment and notice the urge to rush ahead to the next thing.
4. Notice when you make judgments such as "good" or "bad" and "right" or "wrong."
5. Notice the urge to hold on to some feelings (e.g., happiness, calmness) and to push others away (e.g., sadness, worry).
6. Notice the urge to think you already know what something is; instead, try to observe things exactly as they are.
7. Practice accepting that all of these reactions are part of being human.

EXERCISE **Bringing mindful attention to fear and anxiety**

Continue observing and recording your anxious responses in the moments when they occur. Practice bringing the same skills that you use in the breathing mindfulness exercise to monitoring your anxiety. Notice the thoughts, feelings, and sensations that arise with anxiety. Notice the judgments that arise in response. Practice self-compassion, remembering that your responses are part of being human.

5

developing the skills of mindfulness

HOW TO BRING KIND ATTENTION
INTO YOUR DAILY LIFE

Josette walked downstairs in the morning, feeling at ease after her brief mindfulness practice. As she walked into the kitchen, she noticed that Marco had left dirty dishes in the sink—again. She immediately felt frustrated, thinking, "Why can't he put them in the dishwasher like I asked him to?" Her thoughts came quickly: "I need to catch the bus. I don't have time to deal with this right now. I have to get into work and finish up that project. What if I can't get the project done? My boss is going to be so disappointed in me." Her shoulders and neck grew tense, her breath short. Then she noticed the quickness of her emotional response, this spiral in thoughts, and the changes in her body. She took a deep breath and smiled as she rinsed off the dishes before putting them in the dishwasher. It continued to amaze her how quickly her mood could change and her thoughts could cascade in response to such a seemingly minor trigger. She noticed the warm water on her skin as she looked at the dishes, remembering the fun she and Marco had had picking them out before they moved in together. As she waited for the bus, she thought about all the things Marco did to keep the house in order

and thought perhaps it was OK for her to be the one who did the
dishes most of the time.

Josette's experience illustrates how regularly practicing mindfulness can help us notice our reactions and the ways our stress can spiral. Mindfulness practice won't keep us from having anxious, frustrated, angry, or sad thoughts and reactions—these are all part of being human. But it may help us notice these reactions as they unfold and keep our reactions from feeding on themselves in an intensifying spiral that gets in the way of our lives and our well-being. If Josette hadn't been able to notice the reactions she was having, her physiological, emotional, and cognitive reactions to the situation would have continued to intensify, making it harder for her to make choices about her actions. In this reactive state, she might have taken actions that actually made her situation worse (e.g., making her later to work, starting a fight with Marco, without any awareness of the positive feelings she also had toward him) and her reactions would interfere with her ability to do things that were important to her (like functioning effectively at work). By seeing the reactions she was having and bringing awareness to them, she was able to stop the escalating spiral and reengage in living her life as she chose to.

The way we told Josette's story made it seem that she shifted into mindful awareness automatically, without effort. She probably did. But only because (1) she had been practicing mindfulness regularly and (2) she, like the rest of us, had an innate capacity to be mindful. Thanks to the self-preservation instincts and cognitive abilities discussed in Chapter 1, steady-state mindfulness is not our habitual way of going through life. Through practice we can tap back into this natural capacity, developing the skill so we can use it during our day the way Josette did.

In this chapter we present a number of different ways to practice and cultivate this skill and address some of the challenges that often come up when we try to bring this new skill into our lives. Later chapters explore how mindfulness can help us use our emotional responses more effectively, turn toward challenging experiences instead of away from them, and live more fulfilling lives. As you develop these skills, you will be able to use mindfulness in the moment the way Josette did.

Weaving mindfulness into your daily activities will weaken the hold anxiety has on your life and allow you to live more freely and fully. But most people find it extremely challenging to invite in frightening worries and uncomfortable physical sensations with an open heart. Cultivating a mindful stance toward one's private experiences is a process that often requires taking a radically new view of anxiety and other emotions while at the same time practicing some of the most essential skills of mindfulness. That's why we start with building and strengthening the foundation skills of mindfulness in everyday, neutral, even boring situations. Once you can do that, using mindfulness in anxiety-provoking or distressing situations becomes much easier.

You might think of the practices in this chapter as the drills and workouts athletes do to prepare for games, where a range of skills needs to be applied more flexibly. And in the same way that these basketball or football practices confer benefits beyond more skillful play on the court or field, you'll see multiple benefits of mindfulness well before you begin using it in highly stressful situations. A wealth of research has demonstrated that practicing mindfulness can improve sleep, reduce physical pain, boost immune system functioning, and increase relationship satisfaction, to name just a few benefits.

Research has shown that mindfulness practice can help to decrease:

- Anxiety
- Insomnia
- Stress
- Risk of coronary heart disease
- Substance use
- Urges to smoke
- Relapse into depression
- Chronic pain
- Symptoms of fibromyalgia

Research has also shown that mindfulness practice can help to improve:

- Quality of life
- Relationship satisfaction and closeness
- Sexual functioning
- Attention
- Immune system functioning

- Skin clearing among those with psoriasis
- Diabetes self-management
- Longevity and health among nursing home residents

Regularly practicing mindfulness can reduce the overall level of stress and anxiety in your life, making it easier to deal with challenges that arise. Another general benefit of mindfulness is that it brings us more closely in touch with the moments of our lives. Practicing mindfulness can transform even the most mundane experiences into cherished moments.

> *Mindfulness not only reduces overall stress and anxiety in your life but also can turn unremarkable experiences into cherished moments.*

Zoe drove home from work with her mind spinning with memories of frustrations from her day and plans for the next several hours. She worked out a plan for making dinner quickly so that she would have time to eat with the kids before heading out for her night class. She kept replaying what she'd said in the meeting at work, wondering whether she was out of line and how her words might come back to haunt her. When she walked into the house, she was greeted by both girls clamoring for her attention while the phone rang. She began absentmindedly gathering ingredients for dinner while she gave the girls instructions to clean their rooms. Then she remembered her commitment to practice mindfulness each day and that she hadn't practiced that morning. She glanced at the clock, did some quick calculations, and decided that she could spare 5 minutes to practice and still make it to class on time. She asked the girls to leave her alone for 5 minutes and settled on the cushion she'd set up in the corner of her bedroom. As she brought her awareness to her breath, her mind continued to race with thoughts of the day and plans for the evening. Again and again, she gently brought her awareness to her breath. She smiled as she noticed how quickly her mind was off and running each time. She felt her shoulders release a bit as her breath deepened and her thoughts slowed down just slightly. When her timer went off, she took one last deep breath and called for the girls to come keep her company in the kitchen. As she prepared their meal, she listened to her daughters tell stories from their day, smiling at their way of seeing events. As the aromas of the meal filled the air, Zoe felt a sense of contentment, enjoying this moment in her day that she might have missed otherwise.

Mindfulness practice can be either formal or informal. Formal practice involves setting aside dedicated time to practice skills on a regular basis. Informal practice involves bringing mindful attention to your internal experiences and your surroundings as you go about your daily activities. Both can help you develop mindfulness skills, in the same way that an athlete benefits from both speed- or strength-building work and scrimmaging.

Beginning a Formal Mindfulness Practice

Formal mindfulness practices are activities that require setting aside some time to practice every day or a few days a week. Mindfulness of breath, which you tried in the last chapter, is considered a formal practice, as are meditation and yoga. Formal practices require you to commit to investing some time in taking care of yourself—no easy feat, given the demands on our time and the pressure to be productive. But formal practices can be extremely beneficial in helping us learn firsthand about the ways our minds work.

Research has demonstrated a correlation between regularly practicing mindfulness and benefiting from it, so we recommend that you commit to spending at least 5 to 10 minutes a day in formal practice. If you want to do more, great. Many people find that a regular mindfulness practice of 15, 25, or 45 minutes is extremely helpful. If you want to do less, we completely understand. And yet we would still ask you to consider making this commitment to yourself. It's OK if it feels uncomfortable because it's not something you usually do, or you're not sure it will help, or it feels like a waste of time. In our experience, it's much easier to make an accurate judgment about whether formal mindfulness practice can benefit you once you've given it a serious try.

Regular formal practice of mindfulness can help us develop this skill so we can use it in our lives. Just like any new habit we try to develop (flossing our teeth, exercising regularly, eating healthily), it's very challenging to add something new to our lives. The more we can make something part of a regular routine, and do it the same way every day, the more likely we are to establish a habit we can keep going throughout our lives.

Tips for Starting a Regular Formal Mindfulness Practice

- Pick a specific time of day for your practice.
  - It's often useful to tie practice to daily activities. So, first thing in the morning, just after your morning shower, before or after lunch, before or after dinner, or before bed is a good option for establishing this new habit.
- Pick a specific place.
  - If possible, pick a place where you aren't likely to be interrupted.
  - Using the corner of a room or facing a wall can be a way to make a space when no separate space is available.
  - Sometimes it can help to put specific things in this space, like pictures on the wall, incense or burning candles, soothing music, or gentle lighting to create an atmosphere that will be associated with your practice. These items become cues for mindfulness practice in the future, helping to strengthen your developing habit.
- Use a timer or an alarm (like on a cell phone) so that you can set the time of your practice and not have to track the time.
  - The most important thing is that you practice for the full time you intend to, so it's better to practice for 5 minutes and stay for the full 5 minutes than to plan to practice for 15 minutes but stop after 12. Part of the practice is sticking to the intention no matter how many thoughts and impulses to stop arise.
  - For those who have never tried mindfulness, we often recommend beginning with 5 or 10 minutes of practice and then lengthening the practice if you choose to over time. (If 5 minutes is too challenging at first, start with 1 or 2 minutes and then lengthen your practice.) Other people start with longer periods, like 25 or 30 minutes. Choose whichever approach seems more reasonable to you. Again, some regular practice is better than

an intention to have a longer practice that is never met. Often it is easier to add 5 to 10 minutes to daily routines than to add a longer period.

- Make a commitment to yourself to practice daily for at least a week or two.
  - You (like all of us) have been practicing anxious responding for a long time, so learning new habits will take time and practice. Soon you'll be able to see for yourself how this new practice can help you. But to get to that place, you will need to commit to the practice regularly so you can build up the skill and see its effects.
  - As with any other life change, it can be challenging to get started on a new habit, but it's satisfying to commit to something and find a way to fit it into our lives.
  - All of us can benefit from some time set aside for our own well-being. Think of the practice as something you're doing for yourself, which will also help those around you in time.
- Find strategies to remind yourself of your practice.
  - Always practicing after an already daily ritual, like brushing your teeth or taking vitamins, can help you remember to practice.
  - Visual cues, like colored stickers in visible places, can serve as useful reminders. Placing this book where you'll see it first thing in the morning can help you remember to practice in the morning.
  - Writing practice into calendars is a good way to remember and also to be sure that time is set aside.
- If you're like us, you'll find that every day you come up with reasons **not** to practice. This is natural. Notice the thoughts and practice anyway, to see what it feels like to practice even if you don't feel like it or you have a good reason not to do it.
  - Notice the obstacles that come up—these are probably obstacles that come up in other areas of your life. You might want to start a list of "reasons not to practice" so that you can notice them all and then go ahead and practice anyway.
  - Remember that practicing will often not be enjoyable or comfortable. The goal of this exercise is to spend time bringing your awareness back each time it wanders. There is no way to

this wrong. See the box "Working with Anxiety" (pages 103–104) for more discussion of how practice can be helpful even when it isn't comfortable.

— If you miss a day of practice, be kind to yourself about it and recommit to a daily practice.

— One of the biggest obstacles to changing any habit is how we respond to any failures in our efforts at behavior change. Anyone who has tried to diet or start an exercise routine or quit smoking knows that "slips" or "lapses" are common. The key to successful behavior change is forgiving yourself for these slips and recommitting to goals. Practice this skill with your mindfulness practice. When you forget to do it, take that as an opportunity to find new ways of remembering for the next day.

• Monitor your practice.

— It can be helpful to track your practice. You can start a notebook and just write down each time you practice how long the practice lasted and anything you noticed that you want to remember.

Beginning with the Breath

The most common way to begin mindfulness practice is to focus on the breath, as illustrated in Chapter 4. For many people, focusing on the breath is a lifetime practice. One way to begin is by counting the breath.

After settling into a comfortable, alert, seated position on a cushion or a chair (as described in Chapter 4), begin noticing where you can feel your breath. This may be in your belly, your chest, the back of your throat, or your nostrils. Allowing your awareness to settle on this spot, begin counting your in breaths. Count from 1 to 10 and then count backward back to 1. Each time you notice your attention wander, begin back at 1 again. Your practice may involve counting 1 repeatedly—this is fine. There is no goal of reaching 10.

The counting is simply a way of noticing when your attention wanders. For instance, when you notice yourself counting to 12, that's a pretty good indicator of your mind wandering! Each time your awareness wanders, kindly and gently guide it back to the breath, counting 1 at the in breath. Simply continue with this process until the time you've designated is up. When your timer sounds, take one more breath with awareness as you prepare to return to your daily life.

Encountering Challenges in Mindfulness Practice: Working with Anxiety

Often mindfulness practice will lead initially to an increased awareness of symptoms of anxiety, which can make us feel like things are getting worse instead of better. This can be very discouraging and naturally makes us want to stop practicing. Increased awareness can lead to even more judgments and criticisms ("Why can't I keep my attention on my breath? I am so bad at this!"). Given how used to turning away from discomfort we all are, it is very natural to instinctively stop practicing when this happens. However, if we stick with it, we will find that this initial discomfort often subsides and we become more able to tolerate discomfort and anxiety as we begin to see the ebb and flow of our experience. It takes a bit of a leap of faith to make our way through these initial challenges, which is why we ask you to commit to regular practice for at least a week or two so that you can start to see the range of experiences you can have while practicing mindfulness.

When physical, emotional, or cognitive signs of anxiety arise, bring curious awareness to them, as if you're seeing them for the first time. Allow yourself to really notice what tightness in your chest feels like, or the steady stream of critical thoughts you experience. Bring compassion to yourself for having these challenging experiences. And gently bring your attention back to your breath. This new way of noticing will help to transform your experience if you stick with it.

On the other hand, sometimes people find mindfulness practice extremely relaxing at first, which naturally makes them want to practice more and more. Inevitably, however, this experience will pass and everyone will have a practice with a busy, crowded, anxious mind when feelings of frustration, sadness, or fear arise. This can be very discouraging and could lead you to give up the practice, convinced that it no longer "works." Again, remember that mindfulness is a way of being in our lives, as they are. While it may be pleasant at times, it can also be very useful to experience distress or anxiety during practice. If we can stick with mindfulness practice and continue to pay attention to our experiences even when feeling uncomfortable, we can learn some important information about anxiety and how we respond to it. What we learn will be extremely helpful when we begin to apply mindfulness to anxiety-provoking situations. Practicing with anxiety on the cushion (or chair) makes it easier to continue to live our lives fully when we encounter anxiety in our lives. Also, these experiences give us an opportunity to practice being in the moment in the presence of responses that often pull us out of the moment and out of our lives. As we discuss in Chapter 6, living life fully involves experiencing the full range of emotional experiences. If we're willing to be present in our lives only under certain conditions, we're guaranteed to miss out on much of what life has in store for us.

Breathing from the Belly

Traditional mindfulness practices emphasize allowing the breath to be as it is, without trying to change it. But for those who are struggling with anxiety, we often introduce mindful diaphragmatic breathing as a way of cultivating awareness while also gently slowing down a racing mind. If you want to try this out, take a moment now to breathe as you do normally.

> *Breathing from the diaphragm can help slow down the racing mind that is part of anxiety.*

Do you feel your breath in your chest more than your belly? Interestingly, as infants we start out by breathing in the belly, but over time many of us begin breathing primarily in our chest. It is very common to breathe more from the chest when we feel like we need to get a lot of things done or like there is a threat present. This kind of breathing activates our sympathetic nervous system, which is great if we need to run or fight, but is less helpful when the tasks in front of us involve something less active. Although these reactions and this activation are usually automatic, we can also shift our breathing on purpose and activate our parasympathetic nervous system, the system that helps us recover from this kind of stimulation.

Take a moment now and put your hand on your belly. See if you can breathe into your belly, allowing the breath to travel through your chest and down to your belly and then back out the same way.

You may notice that this feels awkward or that you feel some tension in your body as you breathe this way. This is very common for people who tend to breathe more shallowly from their chests on a regular basis. This new, deeper type of breath takes practice to get used to. Don't push yourself too hard— just invite your breath to slow down a little bit, to become a little bit deeper. And if it remains more shallow, that's OK too. If you notice that trying to slow your breath down makes you feel more stressed, just shift back to noticing your breath and counting it, as described above.

Zoe had been practicing mindfulness for several weeks and really enjoying the changes she was noticing in her quality of life. She found herself enjoying her time with her friends and family more, and her work seemed more fulfilling to her. Because her practice seemed so helpful, she found it very easy to make time for it. One day she noticed she was feeling particularly agitated before she sat down to practice. She was angry with a coworker and anxious about an ongoing project that wasn't going well. She anticipated the relief she would feel after her practice and happily sat down and began to focus on her breath. As always, her mind was busy. She gently brought her awareness back to her breath, time and

time again. She waited for the sense of peace and grounding she so often experienced in her practice, but it did not come. She began to wonder what she was doing wrong and to try harder to be mindful, compassionate, and accepting. Her mind became busier, and her feeling of agitation increased. She thought, "Why can't I do this right?" She wondered whether she wasn't good enough at mindfulness to make it "work" when she really needed it. She noticed how uncomfortable she felt sitting and hoped her time would be up soon. Then she remembered something she'd read about accepting things as they were, even if they weren't pleasant. She smiled, realizing that in her efforts to be "mindful" she was criticizing herself and her practice and demanding that it be other than it was. She spent the remainder of her practice noticing her feelings of agitation and her feelings of disappointment that relief wasn't coming. She felt compassion for herself. Although her agitation didn't go away, being able to see it clearly made it seem less menacing and destructive. She went through the rest of her day appreciating the new lessons she had gained from her practice that day.

Mindfulness Skills

By practicing mindfulness regularly, we develop a number of skills that will help us live the lives we want to be living:

AWARENESS

- Increasing the ability to notice where our attention is, how often it shifts, gently bringing it back to the focus.
- Expanding awareness so it captures the fullness of our experience. Anxiety often narrows our awareness to potential threats; mindfulness can expand our awareness so that we notice other aspects of a situation, other sensations, and other emotions.

PRESENT MOMENT

- Gently bringing the mind back to right here, right now, as we sit on the cushion, breathing in and breathing out, whenever the mind moves to memories of the past and plans or worries for the future.

SELF-COMPASSION

- Often the thoughts that arise while we're practicing are judgments or criticisms: "Why can't I just count to 10? I'm terrible at this. I'm never going to learn to do it. I'm wasting my time here." When we notice these thoughts arising, we can practice having compassion for ourselves and our experience. It's important not to judge our judging, though. Judging and criticizing are natural and often become a habit. We can notice this pattern and feel compassion for this struggle without criticizing ourselves for doing it.

BEGINNER'S MIND

- During our practice, we can greet each observation of our breath and each distraction as if it were our first time noticing it. This "beginner's mind" perspective helps us see things fully, as they are, instead of as we expect them to be. We may notice that each practice is different—sometimes our mind is moving very quickly from one thought to the next, and sometimes it's more settled. We can notice each of these states as they are, rather than expecting things to be the way they were the day before.

ACCEPTING THINGS AS THEY ARE

- A very common experience during any type of mindfulness practice is noticing experiences that seem desirable (e.g., a sense of calmness or relaxation or peace) and those that seem less desirable (e.g., a busy mind, sensations of tension, a string of worries). Repeated practice helps us greet each of these experiences as part of our practice. A busy, worried mind is just what is here right now. It is not inherently better or worse than a peaceful mind. It is just the way things are in a given moment. When we respond to it that way, we can reduce the reactivity that comes from wishing that things were other than they are. We can learn to approach whatever comes up with gentleness. Having this experience repeatedly, while we practice, can help us accept whatever arises in our daily lives, including the inevitable worries and stressors we face during the day.

- Accepting things as they are is not the same thing as resignation. We may accept that things are as they are and then choose actions with the intention of making changes (as we describe in later chapters). Josette, at the beginning of this chapter, might accept that Marco is not good at putting dishes in the dishwasher and yet still decide that she wants to try to find a way to encourage him to be better at doing this because this change is important to her. Similarly, we might recognize having a busy, stressed mind, accept that this is how things are in a given day, and decide we want to make changes in our lives to reduce the frequency of this state of being (for instance, cutting down our workload or adding more frequent mindfulness practice to our lives).

Mindfulness of Sounds

After practicing regularly for a week or two, you may want to start trying out some new types of formal mindfulness practice. It's also fine to continue using the breath as a focus and make that your regular practice. You can either keep counting or move to just using the breath as an anchor and keep bringing your awareness back to your breath each time it wanders.

You may decide to try a slightly different practice. One that we often use is mindfulness of sounds (adapted from Zindel Segal, Mark Williams, and John Teasdale's mindfulness-based cognitive therapy). You can read it below and practice it on your own, or go to the book website (listed in the Introduction, page 5) and download an audio recording to listen to while you practice. Often, recordings can be particularly helpful when you first learn a practice, although we also encourage you to practice at times without the recording so that you fully develop your own skills without relying solely on the recordings.

Begin your practice the same way you begin mindfulness of breath—noticing how you are sitting and gently bringing your awareness to your breath. After a few moments of focusing on your breath, allow the focus of your awareness to shift from your breath to your ears. Begin allowing your awareness to open and expand from your ears so that you notice sounds as they arise, wherever they arise. Rather than searching for sounds, or trying to listen for particular sounds, do your best to simply open your mind to any sounds that arise, from any and all directions. You may notice sounds that are close or sounds that are far away, sounds that are in front of you or behind you, to the side, above, or below. Allow your awareness to extend to all the sounds around you. You may notice obvious sounds and also subtle sounds.

While you allow your awareness to take in these sounds, try to be aware of sounds simply as sensations. You may notice that you begin thinking about the sounds, labeling them, or judging them. Each time that happens, reconnect instead, as best you can, with direct awareness of their sensory qualities—their pitch, timbre, volume, and duration, rather than their meanings or implications.

Each time you notice that your awareness has wandered away from sounds in the moment, gently acknowledge this and guide your attention back to the sounds as they arise and pass from one moment to the next, noticing judgments as they arise and gently coming back to your awareness of sound as it is.

Suki practiced mindfulness of sounds and found that when she heard noises she quickly labeled and judged them—the sound of a truck backing up was labeled annoying; the sound of a bird singing was beautiful, and she felt disappointed when it stopped. Repeated practice helped her notice that it was very difficult to hear sounds in her environment simply for their pitch and volume. Instead, she noticed, her mind quickly and naturally labeled the source of the sound, judged the sound, and wanted more of certain sounds and less of others, and she began to see how these tendencies led her to feel dissatisfied with things as they were. As she cultivated awareness of sounds as they were—the pitch and timbre, instead

of the meaning attached to them—she found that she could greet each sound with beginner's mind just noticing it, rather than feeling drawn toward or away from it. She also began using this skill in other areas of her life—seeing how she immediately judged things as desirable or undesirable (e.g., traffic on the way to work or a moment of silence while her son slept). When she practiced just experiencing each thing as it occurred, without becoming wrapped up in wanting more or less of it or thinking about how awful or wonderful it was, she found she was able to respond to events (like her son waking up unexpectedly) with less stress and reactivity.

Encountering Challenges in Mindfulness Practice: Nothing Is Happening!

During your practice you may notice the thought that nothing is happening and this practice cannot possibly be useful. You're not alone! The process of mindfulness is slow, and the changes that occur are subtle and unfold over time. So it's easy to feel like practicing mindfulness isn't doing anything and to give up the practice. Often the practice itself is experienced as boring. Our minds are filled with alternative activities that would be more enjoyable or useful than spending time sitting still and noticing our breath. Yet learning how to remain engaged in our lives even with feelings of boredom can be a valuable experience, as is learning how to watch feelings of boredom rise and fall. Most of us spend some of our time doing something other than what we most feel like doing in a given moment. Having the opportunity to notice what thoughts and feelings arise as we engage in a task that is not immediately appealing can help us learn to do the things in our lives that are boring or unsatisfying in the short term yet are tied to things that matter to us (such as playing Candyland for the twentieth time, which brings great joy to a child but great boredom to an adult). Bringing patience to our practice can help us stick with it so that we can start to see how it can enhance our lives, and it also allows us to develop our skill of patience, which we can use in other areas of our lives.

A metaphor that we sometimes use to capture the experience of doing something that seems boring or undesirable in service of something else comes from Jamail Yogis's *Saltwater Buddha*. He describes a realization he has while surfing: When you spend the day surfing, the goal is to spend time standing on your board, riding a wave. However, a large part of your day will be spent "paddling out" so that you are in a good position when the next wave comes in. Although no one goes surfing out of a desire to spend time paddling out, this paddling out is an essential part of the process of surfing. In a similar way, if we want to be more fully engaged in our lives and be able to notice our reactions and choose our actions, spending time in formal meditation can be very helpful, even if it seems in the moment like we aren't doing anything. And practicing doing something that seems boring or useless, regardless of the thoughts we have or the impulses we have to stop, can help us when we're in our lives and there's some "paddling out" to be done, like studying for an exam that will help us pursue a meaningful career or going on a lot of first dates so that we can eventually make a romantic connection with someone.

Javid started a regular mindfulness practice because he had read that it might help him with his anxiety. He made a commitment to sitting every morning for 15 minutes and following his breath. He kept to his regular schedule and practiced every day for a week. He found the practice extremely challenging. He felt like he spent the entire time losing his focus on his breath. He noticed every pain and ache in his body and also every anxious thought that went through his head and every anxious sensation in his body. He repeatedly had thoughts about all the work he had to do and an impulse to get up and do his work instead of sitting. Other people he knew talked about feeling relaxed when they practiced; he wondered why he didn't have that experience. He kept thinking about stopping, yet he kept practicing even though he couldn't see any changes in his anxiety. Then, one day during his practice, he noticed that his mind had wandered off into worries about the future. And for a moment he was able to see that those worries were thoughts he was having, not accurate predictions or dire warnings, as they seemed to be. He smiled as he brought his attention back to his breath, amazed at how quickly his mind was able to jump to catastrophic predictions. He experienced a moment of peace and calm. It vanished quickly, as his mind wandered again. Yet having that experience showed him the kind of change that was possible. He went to work feeling more hopeful than he had in years.

Mindfulness of Physical Sensations

Often people who experience anxiety experience a lot of physical sensations and have strong reactions to these sensations. It can be helpful to practice mindful awareness of these sensations as a different way of responding to the sensations that naturally occur. Read the exercise below and then take a moment to practice it before reading on. This is one of many practices that you might find helpful to use occasionally as you develop a regular schedule of formal mindfulness practice.

Begin by closing your eyes or looking down and settling in your chair so that you are upright but comfortable, noticing the way you are sitting ... the way your body feels in the chair ... the places where your body is touching the chair. Notice your breath and where you feel it in your body and just allow your awareness to expand so that you notice any sensations that arise in your body—tension or soreness in your muscles, the feeling of the air on your skin, sensations of hunger, any physical sensations that arise. ... Notice sensations as they arise, without labeling or judging them, just noticing them as they are—"a sense of tension here," "a feeling of coldness here"—and if judgments arise, noticing these too and shifting awareness back to your body, to the sensations you are experiencing, allowing each sensation to be, as it is, for however long it remains, just noticing it and continuing with expanded awareness.

This practice can help you get into contact with the responses in your body. As we said in Chapter 1, anxiety often affects our bodies, making our muscles tense or sore or leaving us feeling jittery. And when we notice these sensations in our body, we often respond with judgments about them: "Why am I anxious again? Why can't I just relax?" By practicing noticing our sensations in a compassionate way, we can start to interrupt this spiral in our daily lives.

> *If we can break the habit of automatically scratching when we feel itchy, can we break the habit of automatically avoiding when we feel afraid?*

Encountering Challenges in Mindfulness Practice: Physical Discomfort

The act of sitting still for a period time often brings with it physical sensations such as soreness in the neck, back, shoulders, or legs or limbs falling asleep. Any consistent experience of pain should be addressed by altering your position, for instance, adding an extra pillow or moving your hands from your lap to rest on each leg (which may reduce shoulder pain). More transient experiences that don't indicate any physical risk, such as limbs falling asleep or itchy skin, however, present an interesting opportunity.

Typically, we make some sort of adjustment in response to these physical sensations, without much thought. But what if we didn't? What if we responded to an itch by noting with gentle awareness the physical sensation along with all the thoughts and impulses that arise in response to the sensation, such as "If I don't scratch my leg, I'm going to go crazy"? Mindfulness might reveal to us that thoughts and impulses don't always have to be followed. Noticing impulses without automatically responding is, in fact, an incredibly valuable skill to apply to more challenging areas of our lives. Not always reacting reflexively to internal urges and impulses gives us more choices about our actions.

At first it can be difficult not to respond to an itch or other discomfort because we often assume that such sensations will grow stronger and eventually become unbearable if we don't take some action to relieve them. Interestingly, that is not always the case. Sometimes if we carefully observe a reaction rather than fighting against it or impulsively responding to it, its frequency and intensity may change in ways that surprise us. Simply noticing an itch can at first make us even more aware of the discomfort. Yet bringing patient and curious attention to itchiness may reveal that sensations often ebb and flow.

Just to be clear, being mindful doesn't mean you can never choose to scratch an itch, stretch a muscle, or, for that matter, avoid an anxiety-provoking conversation (even authors and researchers in the field of mindfulness and anxiety do these things from time to time). But being mindful allows us to recognize the frequency with which we respond automatically to events and experiences without acknowledging the full range of choices available to us and gives us an opportunity to choose our actions instead. We talk more about this in the following chapters.

Mindfulness-Based Progressive Muscle Relaxation

Another practice that expands our awareness of our physical sensations is mindfulness-based progressive muscle relaxation, or MB-PMR. This mindfulness exercise is adapted from a procedure called *progressive muscle relaxation*, or PMR, which involves systematically tensing and releasing different muscle groups in the body. There are two goals of this exercise. The first is to learn how to notice subtle cues of tension in different parts of your body. For example, people often don't notice tension across their shoulders and back until it is so tight their shoulders have crept all the way up to their ears and only a professional massage therapist could work the kinks out! Mindfulness helps us become aware of earlier, more subtle cues of tension that are easier to respond to. This brings us to the second goal of the exercise: to learn to release that tension. MB-PMR is based on the principle of a pendulum—pulling it in one direction and releasing it allows the pendulum to swing farther in the other direction than simply pushing it would. In a similar way, tensing slightly and releasing can start the momentum toward deeper muscle relaxation.

Something important to keep in mind if you try MB-PMR is that you should spend only 5 seconds or so tensing each muscle group, and the tension should be very slight and gentle. Sometimes people do this practice with such intensity that they end up tensing their muscles a lot, and that's not what we're working toward! You shouldn't feel pain, just the sensation of tension. You can read the instructions below and then practice this exercise on your own.

For this practice, you may want to sit in a comfortable, reclining chair or lie on the floor so that you are using as few of your muscles as possible. You can also do it sitting as you do for other practices, but being in a position where your whole body is fully supported helps. Begin by bringing your awareness to your breath and then to sensations in your body. After a few moments, bring your awareness to the muscles in your neck, noticing any tension you feel there. Then, by lowering your head toward your chest or pushing your head back against the chair or floor, bring a slight tension into your neck for a few seconds. Now release all the tension, allowing the chair or floor to fully support your head and neck as you breathe gently and notice what it feels like to let your neck muscles lengthen and smooth out. Allow that process to continue for 30 seconds or more. Then tense those muscles again for 5 seconds and release them for 45 seconds or so, just allowing these muscles to continue to lengthen. Next, bring your awareness to the muscles in your shoulders and upper back. By pushing your shoulders up or back, tighten those muscles and notice what that feels like. Then release, sinking into the chair, allowing the muscles in your shoulders and upper back to relax more and more. Bring your awareness to any sensations in your body as you let any tension in that area drain away. After 30 seconds or so, repeat the process of tensing briefly and then releasing for 45 seconds or so. Then scan the rest of your body and see if you notice any tension in other parts of your body—your face (particularly your jaw), your arms, hands, legs, feet. If you do, bring your awareness to those muscles, briefly tense them, and then release them, paying attention to what it feels like to allow those muscles to continue to relax, more and more. Repeat this process and then allow all the muscles in your body to continue lengthening and smoothing out.

If you find MB-PMR helpful and you're interested in practicing it more extensively, we've provided several recordings of the procedure on the book website. The most extensive one involves 16 muscle groups and can take up to 45 minutes. Daily practice is strongly recommended. But over time, you can reduce to the seven-muscle-group version, and eventually a four-muscle-group version, so that it takes less and less time to move through your body and relax it.

Adding Movement

Although formal mindfulness practice often involves sitting still, you can also practice mindfulness while moving. One practice that you might want to try is walking mindfully.

Find a place where you can easily walk in a circle and won't feel self-conscious about moving slowly and with intention. Begin by bringing your awareness to where your feet are touching the ground and what it feels like to hold your body up. Allow your awareness to settle briefly on your breath, noticing what it feels like to breathe in and out while standing. Now, while you inhale, slowly raise one foot, noticing what it feels like to lift it off the ground. While exhaling, place the foot back on the ground and shift your weight onto it. Repeat this process with your other foot. Continue to walk slowly, taking a single breath with each step, continually bringing your awareness back to the sensations in your body as you engage in this simple, usually automatic, movement.

Gentle yoga is another opportunity for mindful movement. Yoga classes or videotapes provide an excellent opportunity for cultivating mindful awareness while also moving your body. Yoga provides an excellent opportunity for noticing our judgments—so often we have thoughts like, "Why can't I stretch further? The person next to me is better at this than I am. I'm so out of shape. Yesterday I was so much more flexible." These are the same kinds of thoughts that occur to us as we do other things in our lives: "I wish I were funny like Tony." "Why can't I meet new people?" "I'm so bad at housekeeping. I used to be better at this." By noticing these thoughts in the context of yoga practice, we can bring compassion to our experience and our attention back to our intention to do something that is healthy for us, regardless of our performance or anyone else's. This experience can make it easier for us to bring similar compassion to these judgmental thoughts as they occur in other aspects of our lives. Other types of intentional movement such as tai chi can also provide excellent opportunities for this kind of practice.

Encountering Challenges in Mindfulness Practice: Finding Time

Chances are you didn't pick up this book because you felt like you had a lot of extra time. Anxiety is usually accompanied by a sense of not having enough time to do everything that needs to be done. We certainly struggle with the same feeling. However, we've discovered repeatedly in our own lives that taking 15 minutes to practice mindfulness leaves us more productive in the rest of our daily tasks and feeling more rewarded by our experiences throughout the day. Practicing regularly allows us to spend less of the day caught up in frustration or annoyance, provides us with more cognitive flexibility for problem solving, and reduces our time spent procrastinating. Even though we learn this repeatedly, we often have to try it out again because it is such an easy lesson to forget. Try for yourself: commit to practicing for a week and see what you notice about how the rest of your day goes.

Also, no matter how overscheduled your day may seem, you

probably spend some time doing things that you don't value highly. Many of our clients have found that they can carve out some time for practice by choosing to play one computer game rather than 10 in a row or watching 15 minutes less TV at night while still watching their favorite shows. Or sometimes asking a partner to watch the children for 15 minutes each evening can provide the window needed for regular practice. If none of these suggestions work, try to practice for 2 minutes a day instead and see how that goes.

Realistically, sometimes people's lives do not easily allow for formal practice. Roxanne had a 6-month-old daughter and a 3-year-old son. Although she tried to set aside time to practice mindfulness regularly, she often found that her daughter would wake up just as she settled on the cushion or her son would come into her room and want her attention. At first she judged herself for not being able to make time for practice and feared that this would mean that the mindfulness-based therapy she was trying wouldn't be helpful. Her therapist suggested that instead she accept that formal practice wasn't fitting into her life in this moment and that she commit to regular informal practice, such as practicing mindfulness while breast-feeding her daughter, showering, folding laundry, and doing dishes. Through these practices, Roxanne noticed how easily her mind moved to the future, to lists of things she had to do and worries about her children. As she developed the ability to turn her attention toward the task at hand, she found she was also able to notice the judgmental thoughts that arose in her interactions with her mother, sisters, and partner and found herself more able to practice compassion in these contexts, reducing her stress and reactivity. Although some formal practice can be extremely useful, this kind of regular informal practice can also help with learning new skills that will help with the cycle of stress and anxiety. So, if you find that despite your best efforts over several weeks you can't establish a formal practice, stick with informal practice for now and keep following along with the book. Maybe you'll take up a formal practice after you experience some of the ways that mindfulness can help you.

Informal Practice

Formal practice acquaints us with our habitual ways of responding (e.g., attention is pulled in multiple directions, thoughts are often judgmental and critical, behaviors are automatic and impulsive) and helps us develop fundamental mindfulness skills. It is equally important that we bring these practices directly to our daily experiences.

Informal mindfulness practice involves purposely bringing your attention to an everyday life activity, like taking a shower or petting your dog. It doesn't require any additional time; the key is to gently bring a new quality of attention to whatever activity you are already engaged in. Informal mindfulness involves approaching a task that is common and mundane with the curiosity of someone who is doing it for the very first time (instead of mindlessly multitasking). For instance, even if you've brushed your teeth more than 21,000 times (twice a day for the last 30 years), imagine doing such a strange thing for the first time. Take a close look at the bristles of the brush—the various lengths of each individual thread, any pattern of wear. Notice the consistency and smell of the paste as you spread it onto the brush, really examining the size, shape, and color of the minty crystals embedded in the gel or paste. Deeply inhale the smell of the paste before you put the brush into your mouth and notice what happens. Do your eyes water slightly? Does it clear your sinuses? Listen to the sound of the brush as it moves across your teeth. Notice any differences in sensitivity across different teeth. Feel the sensation of the water and paste mixing as you go to rinse and notice the strong urge to spit before you actually do so. You can bring this type of observation to virtually any activity during your day. Some suggestions are listed below.

To see what it's like to do something mindfully, pick one of the tasks listed in the box below, or something else you do every day, and spend this week doing it mindfully. Again, you may want to keep a journal or make some notes each time you engage in this informal practice, noticing what it is like for you. At the end of the week, add another daily activity to your practice. See what you notice as you bring awareness to different kinds of activities. You may find that some are often very pleasant, while others are uncomfortable as you notice how difficult it is to maintain awareness or how busy and crowded your mind feels. Remember that challenging practices are also important aspects of your learning, so make sure you don't choose only more "pleasant" types of practice. Each practice brings its own lessons. All practices help to increase flexibility and develop this new habit, while reducing the habit of responding automatically, with attention on the past or future and judgments continually arising.

Just Some of the Activities You Can Do Mindfully

- Eating
- Sitting
- Walking
- Washing dishes
- Folding laundry
- Doing housework
- Taking a shower
- Petting your dog
- Brushing your teeth

- Talking on the phone
- Driving
- Riding the bus or subway
- Cooking
- Listening to music
- Hugging someone
- Working
- Listening to a friend

The ideas and suggestions in the following chapters are based on our own experiences as well as our experiences with clients who have come to us with a range of anxiety symptoms and stressors. By developing your own practice and enhancing your awareness of your experience, you will be able to see how the observations we and others have made fit with your own experiences and apply best to your life. These practices are therefore an important part of how you can make the best use of this book and develop your own mindful path through your anxiety. Now that you have been practicing mindfulness for a little bit, you may find it helpful to do a brief practice before you begin reading each of the following chapters. Just taking a few moments to notice your breath and the way you are sitting in your chair will help you focus fully on the material and see the way it fits your experience.

Encountering Challenges in Mindfulness Practice: Not Being in the Mood to Practice

We and our clients often find that certain mood states seem like reasons not to practice. The thoughts "I'm too tired to practice," "I'm too stressed out and cranky to practice," and "I'm too sad to practice" arise in all of us. At first these seem like reasonable conclusions—many activities seem less appealing when our physical or mental state seems to be off in some way. Wouldn't it be better to practice mindfulness when we're in the right state of mind?

We'll revisit the problems associated with waiting for the right mood or state of mind to act, but many of our clients have passed up promotions or turned down relationships because they didn't feel calm or confident enough to take advantage of the opportunities. Even though it may sound odd at first, practicing mindfulness when you're in a bad mood or tired can also present a wonderful opportunity to practice turning toward things that you habitually turn away from. As we discuss in depth in the next chapter, internal states that we have all learned to ignore, suppress, or avoid often have a great deal to teach us. In addition, the act of turning away from them doesn't always bring relief and, in fact, often makes them more challenging and distressing.

So, each time we notice a tendency to skip practice because of our emotional or physical state, we have a new chance to practice turning toward these experiences and proceed with our practice nonetheless. While practicing, we can welcome the many opportunities to practice responding to our thoughts and feelings with gentleness and openness instead of reactivity and judgment. Exercises in the next few chapters will help you develop these skills.

EXERCISE **Mindful monitoring of fear and anxiety**

Continue mindfully observing and recording your anxious responses in the moments when they occur. Remember, mindfulness involves becoming fully aware of the thoughts, feelings, physical sensations, and images that you experience. Also, observe these reactions with curiosity and interest. View your responses as they are instead of what you know or fear them to be. Notice the pull to label, judge, and react to your anxiety and practice acknowledging that the reactions we have are part of being human.

6

befriending your emotions

Dex came home from work feeling agitated and uneasy. He turned on the TV and flipped through the channels, looking for something to settle his attention on. After watching a show for a few minutes, he would get bored and change the channel again. He went to the kitchen to find something to eat, brought a bag of chips back to the living room, and started watching TV again. He noticed a feeling of heaviness in his chest as he kept munching on chips. His mind kept shifting from things he should be doing to things he wished he'd done before he left work. He noticed his shoulders were tight and hunched as he tried once again to focus on the TV program he was watching. He wished he could just settle down and relax. The more he tried to find something to focus his mind on, the more his mind seemed unfocused. Then he remembered the mindfulness exercises he'd read about. He decided he might as well try to focus on his breath for a few minutes. He put the chips away and turned off the TV and tried to gently bring attention to his breath. Although his mind continued to wander, he brought it back to the breath over and over again. After a few minutes, a wave of sadness came over him, and he began to think about his father, who had passed away earlier that year. He immediately noticed an urge to return to the TV and a craving for more chips. He noticed these responses and stayed with his breath as the sadness continued to emerge, along with images of his father. After several more minutes he noticed a desire to call his sister and talk about their father. He chose to fol-low this impulse. His sister was happy to hear from him, and they both shared their memories and the things they missed about their father. When Dex got off the phone, his sadness was still there, but he also felt a renewed connection to his sister and to the happiness he had felt from being with his father while he was alive. The feeling in his chest was lessened, although still present. The biggest change was that he felt less agitated and uneasy.

Often when people begin practicing mindfulness, they find they enjoy bringing their awareness to their sensory experiences, like notic-ing smells, sounds, and sensations while they eat, shower, or walk out-side. They may also enjoy mindful awareness of experiences like play-ing with a child or spending time with friends. They may also notice that bringing their awareness to emotions of happiness and satisfaction can enhance these emotional experiences. Yet when feelings of sad-ness, fear, anger, or shame arise, awareness no longer seems like such a good idea and often distraction seems more appealing. This is a natural human response to painful emotions; however, gentle, compassionate awareness of our pain reduces our agitation and reactivity and helps us live more fulfilling lives.

Becoming Familiar with Our Emotional Experiences

We all have times when our hearts race, our breath gets shorter, and we experience the emotion of fear, sensing danger and feeling an urge to run or flee. We also have times when our bodies feel heavy and a wave of sadness overcomes us, and we feel like we might cry and like any activity would be too much to take on. At other times we may feel our faces get hot as anger arises and we want to yell at someone or throw something

> *Often our emotions alarm us because we want to avoid acting the way these emotions make us feel like acting.*

because we feel we've been wronged in some way. Often these emotions alarm us and we want to try to feel differently, partly because we want to avoid acting the way these emotions make us feel like acting.

EXERCISE **Exploring the power of emotion**

Take several moments now to think of the last time you felt a strong emotion. After you finish reading this exercise, close your eyes and see if you can picture yourself in the moment when the strong emotion arose. Remember what it felt like in your body, what thoughts you had at the time, and what you felt like doing (and what you did) when you were feeling the emotion. Also, pay attention to any emotions, sensations, or thoughts you have while doing this exercise. Jot down the emotions, bodily sensations, thoughts, and actions/impulses you originally had, as well as those that came up in the exercise.

The first thing you may have noticed when you did this exercise is how strongly the emotions can return just from your trying to remember them. Just recalling an anxious experience can make us feel jittery. Thinking back on an argument can make us angry even though it happened in the past. Often this "emotional recall" is most obvious in the way we feel the emotions in our bodies. Our shoulders can tense up just thinking of something we're worried about; our bodies feel heavy when we remember something sad.

You may also have noticed how the emotions and bodily sensations are so closely tied to thoughts in our head and to impulses to act (or to remain inactive). Being scared usually involves feeling the emotion of fear, thinking worrisome thoughts, experiencing increased pulse rate and respiration, and having the urge to escape. Emotional responses involve a full body and mind response so that thoughts and feelings and actions all feed one another, often making one another more intense and, in the case of distressing emotions, increasing our motivation to try not to feel what we're feeling.

Did you also notice that you didn't want to feel the emotions associated with this memory? It's very common for us to immediately, without even thinking about it, try to get rid of sad, angry, or frightened feelings. Sometimes we can easily distract ourselves and the uncomfortable feelings go away. More often, trying to get rid of emotions can actually make them more distressing and harder to get rid of, as we explore in the next few chapters. For now, just notice

Trying to get rid of emotions can just make them feel worse and make them stick around.

how easy it is to respond to emotions with a desire to avoid them or get rid of them.

You may even have found it hard to think of a time when you felt intense emotions. Or maybe you were aware of a time when you felt strong emotions, but you couldn't figure out exactly what you were feeling. Often we spend so much time trying not to feel our emotions—or we're taught not to talk about how we're feeling—that we end up not really knowing what our emotions are. Have you ever had any of these experiences?

- Are you sometimes aware that you feel "distressed" or "unsettled" but can't tell whether you're sad, scared, ashamed, or angry, or possibly some combination of these responses?
- Does it seem like all you really experience is the anxiety, apprehension, or worry with which you respond to your emotions—to the point where you can't tell what emotional response came before that worry?
- Do you experience a sense of numbness that makes it seem like you aren't having any emotional responses at all?

All of these experiences are natural responses that can occur for a number of reasons. For all of them, bringing gentle awareness to your internal experience will help expand your sense of what your emotional responses are.

Why Do We Have Emotions?

We've seen how emotions are tied to responses in our bodies, thoughts, and urges to act, as well as how we can bring these emotional experiences back just by remembering an event. Why do we have emotions that overtake us this way?

- ***Emotions communicate important information to us and to others.*** An emotional response like fear or anger tells us something about our environment. Fear tells us that we perceive a threat, anger tells us that we've been wronged in some way, and sadness tells us we've lost or lack something we value. The automatic facial and behavioral expressions of our emotions tell others about these experiences as well. A mother's look of horror efficiently teaches her children about a threat in the environment. Angry gestures inform our loved ones that they have done something to upset us and have an opportunity to make amends. These forms of nonverbal emotional communication are more efficient and effective than verbal communication. We pay attention to and remember information better when emotions are

> *Messages delivered with strong emotion get through to us more than any words.*

involved—a fact known not just by psychologists but by many whose business it is to communicate. Advertising agencies, notably, spend billions of dollars to produce commercials that bring us to tears, surprise us, or elicit uncontrollable laughter.

- *Emotions organize and prepare us for action.* The physical sensations and impulses that accompany our emotional responses prepare us to take action in response to whatever has elicited our response. As we discussed in Chapter 1, fear mobilizes us to fight or flee. The rush of adrenaline associated with anger helps us prepare to confront the person who has wronged us. The lethargy associated with sadness allows us to withdraw from other activities so that we can grieve a loss. Emotions also provide signals that can help us improve our lives: anger and sadness can tell us we need to make some kind of change to live a more satisfying life. Even though we all know how anxiety can get in the way of our lives, a moderate amount of anxiety can motivate us to study for an exam, train for a sporting event, or prepare for a presentation.

- *Emotions deepen our experience of life.* It's easy to see how emotions like pride, happiness, and joy enhance our experience of life. But even so-called negative emotions, like sadness, are part of a full life. Can we really experience the joy of being with someone we love without also experiencing the sadness of his or her absence? Often sadness and fear help bring us close to other people as we share our vulnerabilities with those closest to us. And experiencing painful emotions can help us develop empathy for other people's pain and allow us to learn and grow. Although feelings of sadness or fear often feel in the moment like a sign of weakness, as we become more used to these feelings and come to honor them as a badge of a meaningfully lived life, we may find that they are a significant source of strength.

Listening to Our Emotions:
The Hot Stove Analogy

Often we want to avoid our painful emotions. On the surface, this seems like a natural and adaptive human response. These emotions are often upsetting and unpleasant, so we will try to distract ourselves by watching TV, eating junk food, drinking, playing computer games, or doing anything else that takes our mind off the pain. Although this makes a lot of sense, we can run into problems when we ignore the signals our emotions are sending us. Think of emotional pain as being similar to physical pain. Most people would agree that physical pain is unpleasant and that trying to avoid it is a good idea. But imagine that you've put your hand on a hot stove. You would be strongly motivated to try to avoid the associated pain—so what could you do?

You could distract yourself from focusing on the pain (as women do during childbirth or people in some cultures do when they attempt to walk on hot coals). Or you could tell yourself that the pain is not really there (what we sometimes refer to as "denial"). Or you could take a really, really strong pain reliever and keep your hand on the stove.

What would happen if you successfully engaged in these avoidance/ distraction techniques? Your hand would be burned severely. What you obviously need to do is remove your hand from the stove.

But removing your hand automatically, without awareness, is not enough to ensure that you never get burned again. If you remove it without paying sufficient attention to the process, you will not have learned what you need to in this situation. To respond wisely you need to:

- Be aware that you're experiencing the pain
- Be aware of what kind of pain you're experiencing
- Be aware that the stove is what is causing the pain
- Be ready to take action

If you don't pay attention to the pain and correctly identify its source, you could end up with other problems. For instance, what if you thought the pain was caused by being in the kitchen, and so you never entered the kitchen again? This might make it difficult for you to nourish yourself, so it would interfere with living a healthy life. Or what if you thought the pain came from the pan instead of the stove? Again, this would make it difficult for you to cook your favorite foods. Even if you correctly identified the burner flame as the problem, you could decide never to cook again to avoid the risk of pain in the future. Although this might seem like a surefire way to avoid pain, in this scenario you've made avoiding pain more important than nourishing yourself, and that choice is likely to bring about other problems.

The stove example may seem extreme, but it's not at all uncommon for us to avoid a situation to elude pain and suffering, only to find that these self-protective measures have narrowed our choices and caused us other discomfort, in the form of sadness and dissatisfaction.

So let's see how this fits in with an emotional example. Imagine that you're experiencing sadness and disappointment because your current job is not fulfilling. That sadness is uncomfortable, so you naturally want to get rid of it. You might spend your evenings zoning out, watching TV alone, trying to "relax," or you might start staying out late at night with friends, drinking and trying to have a good time so that you don't notice you're feeling sad in that area of your life. You might start finding reasons to miss work or daydreaming when you're there. These things all may reduce the pain of the sadness in the moment, but none of them are likely to resolve the problem (and they may create new problems as you start sleeping less, falling behind at work, and running into more conflicts with coworkers).

Instead of channeling your energy into efforts aimed at avoiding or getting rid of the pain, you need first to acknowledge that you're experiencing pain, recognize that the pain is specifically driven by emotions of sadness and disappointment, and realize that sadness is a response to your current work situation. Only this informed and mindful perspective on your emotions will allow you to take the final step and engage in some action that will resolve the situation (e.g., looking for a new job, new challenges in your current job, or some other way to feel satisfied in a job that you don't enjoy).

Although emotional and physical pain are similar in that both give us important signals that can help us live healthy and adaptive lives, emotional responses are often more complicated than physical pain in many ways. Both emotions and physical pain are associated with *action tendencies*, or an impulse to take certain actions when we feel certain emotions or pain. So when we feel fear or anger, we automatically prepare to fight or flee. This happens on a biological level, even if we don't think about taking these actions. And this preparedness and urge to act can feel to us as though we have to take the action that a specific emotion is tied to. In the case of physical pain, the action tendency is often associated with survival, so we want to take the action associated with the pain. However, sometimes we don't want to take the action that we feel urged to take in an emotional state.

> *Dina was on a third date with Cynthia. Dina had been single for several years and knew that she wanted to develop an intimate relationship. She really liked Cynthia and felt like this could develop into a good relationship for her. As she and Cynthia began talking about personal things, Dina felt her chest tighten and her pulse quicken and had an urge to avoid these topics so she wouldn't be exposed to being hurt. She watched Cynthia's face for signals of rejection and thought she saw evidence that Cynthia was judging her as she talked about a low point in her life. Dina felt a strong urge to change the subject or end the date and protect herself. Yet making this kind of connection was important to her, so she chose to remain in this situation.*

Dina noticed the response she was having and correctly identified that she was afraid of social rejection. The action that would address this fear would be to reduce her vulnerability or end the social contact. However, she chose not to follow this urge and instead decided to take the risk and experience the fear. In this case, by being able to turn toward her emotional experience and see all of its nuances, Dina was able to refrain from a habitual response of avoidance (consistent with the action tendency of fear or anxiety) and instead choose a more effective, values-consistent action that could help her live a more fulfilling life.

> *Mindfulness helps us allow the emotional pain that comes with the most meaningful experiences and thus helps us pursue what matters to us.*

Often the things that matter to us, like loving people, forming emotional connections, taking on challenging tasks, or supporting others in pain, bring with them emotional pain. In these cases, living a fulfilling life means that we notice the pain and allow it, rather than trying to make it go away. Mindfulness can help us befriend our range of emotional experiences, making it easier to make these choices and enrich our lives.

Practicing Befriending Our Emotions

Now we are ready to try a more challenging mindfulness exercise. This time we ask that you focus on a time in your life when you felt sad. Choose a time that was not very recent, but also was not in your childhood. On a scale of 1 to 7, with 1 being no sadness, 4 being moderate sadness, and 7 being extreme sadness, pick an event that is a 4 or 5. So pick a time when you felt sad but not overwhelmed by those feelings.

Being mindful in the presence of a strong emotion is more challenging than when we're not feeling an intense emotion, because emotions narrow our focus and we often try to change our feelings, rather than allowing whatever arises to arise. So don't be discouraged if you find this exercise harder than the ones you have tried before. Remember that any experience you have when practicing is useful, even if it isn't enjoyable. There is no right or wrong way to do these practices. This is just a first attempt to bring gentle awareness to your emotional experience.

First, write a brief description of the situation you've chosen in your notebook so that you can begin to get a clear memory of it. Now think about the sensory experiences during this memory. What do you hear, see, smell, and feel during this event? What do you notice in your body?

Now you can either download an audio recording of this practice from the book's website, or read over the following guidelines for the practice. Then close the book and try the practice on your own for 5 to 10 minutes. You will notice that in these exercises we use -ing words, like *noticing*, instead of *notice*. This helps create a sense of these practices as a process of continuing to bring awareness, rather than a sense that you might reach some end state of noticing and be done. It may sound a little odd at first, but you'll get used to the language in time, and we hope it helps you cultivate the sense of mindfulness as an ongoing process. Because being mindful in the presence of strong emotions is more challenging, this is a particularly good exercise to try first with an audio recording to guide you through it.

Beginning by noticing the way you are sitting. Noticing where your body touches the chair or floor. Then gently bringing your awareness to your breath. Noticing where you feel it in your body. Noticing the sensations as you inhale and exhale.

As your awareness settles on this moment, allow your memory of this sad event to arise. Picture yourself in the situation, noticing what you can see, the sounds you hear.

Then begin paying attention to feelings in your body, noticing any tightness in your body. Becoming aware of the thoughts running through your mind. And observing the emotions you feel.

You may notice more than one emotion or that emotions unfold over time.

Attending to any urges to respond to your experience, any desire to avoid your feelings.

Just noticing your experience, bringing curiousness and compassion to what you are experiencing. Observing what happens to you when you are feeling strong emotions, without altering it or judging your experience.

Noticing anytime you are trying to alter or judging your experience and just letting go, refocusing on the experience.

Paying attention to any efforts to push feelings away or efforts to hold on to feelings.

Noticing how your feelings change or ways they don't change.

When your timer goes off, letting the memory go and bringing your awareness again to your breath and the present moment before you open your eyes.

When you complete this practice, note your observations in your notebook.

As we mentioned above, practicing mindfulness of our emotions can be much more difficult than practicing mindfulness of sounds or sensations. Our minds wander even more when intense emotions are present, and judgments often arise repeatedly. Patiently bringing ourselves back to the practice of gentle, compassionate awareness, allowing whatever arises to be there, helps us learn to remain aware of our emotions instead of trying to push them away or criticizing ourselves for having them. When you notice that you're having an intense emotional response during the day, take note of it and then practice being

> ## Common Observations While Practicing Mindfulness of Emotions
> - Hard to stay focused on the event and the emotion(s)
> - Many efforts to distract or avoid
> - Discomfort from emotional experience
> - New emotions emerged that weren't recognized at the time
> - Emotion became less intense and uncomfortable as practice continued
> - Noticed new things about the event
> - Intensity of emotions rose and fell
> - Many judgments came up

aware of the emotions when you have time for a brief practice. See what you notice about the way different emotions feel in your body and the thoughts and urges associated with them. Be patient with yourself during these practices and continue to practice compassion toward your struggles and experiences.

Emotions and Our Valued Directions

In Chapter 2 you did some exercises to help you identify the ways that anxiety has gotten in the way of living the life that matters to you. In this chapter you have spent time exploring different emotional responses and practicing turning toward these experiences, rather than moving away from them. This practice with our emotions is an important part of embarking on a new path toward the life you want to be living because our emotions are tied to what matters to us.

First, emotional responses are often an indication that we're not living the life we want to be living. In the example above of feeling dissatisfied with work, the feelings of sadness were important cues that work wasn't in line with what was most important. Dex, at the beginning of the chapter, experienced sadness, which helped him realize that he wasn't connecting to his sister in a way that would be meaningful for him.

At the same time, emotional responses often get between us and the life we want to be living. As you identified in Chapter 2, anxiety can keep us from pursuing things that matter to us (just as Dina noticed when she was on a date with Cynthia). Our fear of emotional pain often leads us to avoid engaging in actions that would be rewarding and satis-fying, because they would also make us vulnerable.

For both of these reasons, increasing our awareness of our emotional experience can help us determine the direction that will be meaning-ful for us and to pursue actions that will enhance our lives. Becoming aware of emotions and turning toward them may seem overwhelming at the moment. Often our efforts to avoid our emotions and other factors have led us to experience intense and overwhelming emotions that are very challenging to turn toward. However, these *muddy* emotions can become more clear and informative with practice. In the next chapter, we explore how emotions become muddy and identify ways to clarify our emotional responses so that they can provide useful information and to reduce their interference in our lives.

EXERCISE **Befriending your emotions**

To help you begin to practice turning toward your emotions, try a new monitoring exercise for the next week or two. Instead of just noticing signs of anxiety, begin to notice the emotional responses you're having at the time you're experiencing anxiety. Use your notebook to help you do this exercise. Note the date, situation, and any signs of anxiety that you notice, and then write down the emotions you are experiencing. You may find that the first emotions you notice are anxiety and fear, because those are the ones you are most used to noticing. But bring mindfulness to your experience and see if other emotions are occur-ring at the same time. It takes practice to become familiar with our emotional responses, so don't be frustrated if you find that you often are not aware of what you're feeling. Just noticing that you don't know what you're feeling is an important step toward becoming more in tune with your emotional responses. As you notice your emotions, you may find that judgments or criticisms arise. Notice these and continue prac-ticing kindness and compassion toward your experiences. Remember that all emotional responses are a natural part of being human, not a sign of weaknesses or flaws.

7

using mindfulness to clarify
muddy emotions

Nadir woke up late after a restless night's sleep. He quickly got ready for work and skipped breakfast in an effort to make up some time. On his way to work, he was distracted, thinking about everything he had to do when he got to work and how much he didn't like being late. He forgot about the construction on his usual route and did not take the alternate route he had been taking for the past week. He then found himself stuck in very slow-moving traffic and felt his tension and frustration rising. When he finally got to work, his usual parking lot was closed and he had to circle several times before he found a place to park. He raced to his office, annoyed with the people walking slowly in front of him, and slipped into his chair. He impatiently waited for his computer to start up and then opened up his e-mail. He opened an email from a coworker, which contained feedback on a report he had written the week before. He experienced intense anger and resentment at the suggestions and criticisms and began to write an angry reply.

In the last chapter, we explored the ways that our emotions can give us useful information and motivate us to take important actions. But you may find that, like Nadir and many of us, you more often experience emotions that seem intense and out of proportion to what has just happened in your life. One way of thinking about these confusing emotional responses is that rather than being *clear*, or direct responses to the event that has just occurred, they are *muddy*, making them much more complicated to act on. Just like anxiety and worry, muddy emotional responding can become a habit that feeds on itself so that the more muddy our emotional responses are, the more muddy they become and continue to be. During particularly stressful or challenging times in our lives, muddy emotions may become so common that it's impossible to imagine emotional responses giving us useful information. This makes it even more likely that we'll turn away from rather than toward these responses, which makes the cycle continue. In this chapter, we explore ways to stop this cycle so that our emotions can be clarified and less intense and overwhelming.

How Can We Tell When Our Emotions Are Muddy?

Here are a few signs that the emotional responses we're having may be muddy instead of clear:

- Our reactions seem more **intense** than the situation warrants.
- We cannot identify any specific emotions; we just feel **distressed** or **upset**.
- We find our emotions **confusing** or **overwhelming**.
- Our emotional response feels really **familiar**, like maybe this is a way we respond by habit, or is connected to something in the past.
- We feel a strongly **judgmental** or **critical** response to our reaction.
- Our emotional response is very **long lasting**, rather than being specific to what just happened.
- Instead of feeling like we're having an emotional response, we feel like our emotions **define** us or are just **the way we are**.
- We feel like we're **caught up in** or **entangled** in our emotional response.

What Makes Emotions Muddy?

Not Taking Care of Ourselves

Have you ever noticed that when you don't sleep well the night before, you're more likely to get frustrated with your children, angry with your partner, or annoyed by a coworker the following day? You're not alone! One reason that a good night's sleep is so important (and that not getting enough sleep is so aggravating) is that sleeping enough helps us tolerate life's frustrations and prevents intense reactions that seem disproportionate to the events that precipitated them. Similarly, not eating regularly can affect our ability to regulate our emotional responses and make us more susceptible to overwhelming sadness, fear, anger, shame, and other emotional responses. Many behavioral or physical irregularities can have a significant effect on our moods and emotions. Irregular sleep schedules, lack of downtime, low-grade illness, diets high in junk food and low in protein, and hormonal changes all can make our emotional responses more intense and more long-lasting than if we were healthy, rested, and had eaten properly. Nadir's intense response to his colleague likely happened in part because he had not slept well and had skipped breakfast.

Knowing this can be helpful in a few ways.

1. It can help us remember to try to get more sleep or eat well or take care of ourselves in other ways so that our emotions are less likely to be intense and overwhelming.

2. We're more likely to be able to remind ourselves not to take our strong reactions at face value when we know we haven't been able to take good care of ourselves. For me (L. R.), when I haven't slept well, I try to remind myself in the morning that I'm likely to have really strong negative emotional reactions during the day. Then, when those inevitable reactions come up, I tell myself to wait another day before taking any drastic action so that I can see whether my responses are really caused by the situation or are a result of my being overtired and irritable. This simple strategy has kept me from doing things (like responding with anger to my partner or a colleague) that I would later have regretted.

3. Just knowing that our responses are likely to be muddy may help us recognize the muddiness and find clarity underneath our reactions.

Once you've established a mindfulness practice, these periods of poor self-care are excellent opportunities to increase your formal or informal practice to clarify your emotional responses. An early-morning practice can also be a great way of noticing the early indicators that we're going to have a day filled with muddy emotional responses.

Worrying About or Anticipating the Future

Priya was making her way through her to-do list for the day. She called the twins' doctor to make an appointment for their 12-month check-up. The receptionist told her that there weren't any openings available for another 2 months. Priya felt her heart rate increasing as she imagined the various difficulties that might not be detected if the twins couldn't see the doctor until they were 13½ months old. She wondered whether this delay could cause irreparable harm and scolded herself for being such a negligent mother. Priya began thinking of the future doctor's appointments that would be necessary if, in fact, anything were detected in this visit, and how difficult it would be to fit these into her busy schedule. She imagined her boss's response to her request for more days off to attend to these undetected and, to her knowledge, nonexistent health problems and felt tension in her shoulders. Her mind was spinning so fast that she failed to respond to the receptionist, who eventually hung up. Priya began worrying that she would lose the appointment that was available as she redialed the doctor's office.

As we discussed in Chapter 1, it's very common for us to look ahead and think about how something happening right now might affect the future. This can often help us plan or problem-solve. So when Priya is making this appointment, it will be helpful for her to anticipate what she'll need to change in her schedule to take the twins to the doctor. However, this kind of useful thinking ahead can quickly transform into imagining things that might go wrong. That can lead to increases in our anxiety and can lead us to respond to what is happening in the moment as though things have already gone wrong in the future, which is a muddy response.

Being aware that our minds have jumped to the future can help reduce this muddiness. The monitoring you have been doing has been a good start to seeing the kinds of thoughts you have and how quickly and automatically they can come. You may have already noticed times when you were thinking about the future and having anxious responses associated with potential feared future outcomes. We can easily (and quickly) jump to worrying about something four or five outcomes away from where we are in the moment! It's no wonder our anxiety can feel so overwhelming. In later chapters we try some mindfulness exercises that focus specifically on noticing our thoughts—these can also help with this type of muddiness.

"Leftover" Responses

Lola was nervous as she walked into her review meeting with her boss. Her boss had a reputation for making unfair demands on employees and unjustly criticizing them. Everyone said that you should never talk back when she was criticizing you—instead, they advised everyone to smile and thank her for her useful feedback. So Lola did not express any reactions when her boss began to list her supposed flaws and scold her for errors that she never made. Instead, she apologized for making errors and promised that she would do better in the future. Her shift was over, so she went straight home after the meeting. James greeted her when she walking in the door and gave her a hug. Then he mentioned that she had forgotten to return a library book that morning as planned. Lola felt a rush of intense anger and yelled that all he ever did was criticize her. She caught a glimpse of James's confused look as she stormed out of the room.

Just as a focus on the future can lead to muddy emotional responses, events from the past can also make it harder to sort out our emotional responses in the moment. Our responses can be due to leftover emotions in two different ways. Lola experienced one of them: She felt strong emotions in response to a very upsetting event at work but couldn't express them at the time. As a result, she had a very intense response to her partner that seemed out of proportion to what happened in their interaction. We have all had this kind of experience. We leave an interaction stirred up by something that we haven't been able to express because of our relationship to the person involved, or the context in which it happened, or because we didn't realize we were having a response at the time and we find that we have an intense response later to a milder interaction. Sometimes it's easy to make the connection and understand our response, but sometimes too much time has passed and we're preoccupied, so we just find ourselves puzzled by our responses.

Leftover reactions can also happen over a much longer period. Sometimes we carry specific kinds of pain from past important relationships, like our parents or other family members, teachers, friends, or intimate partners. We might have repeatedly had the experience of being criticized, rejected, or shamed. Even though these experiences have not continued into our present lives, sometimes they were so painful and repeated at the time that we find ourselves having similar kinds of responses to other people in our lives. This can happen because someone reminds us of a person from our past.

It can be very hard to recognize when this is happening. One clue is when an emotional response feels familiar or the words we're saying to ourselves are words that someone else used to say to us. Often it takes several weeks or months of practicing awareness of our emotional responses before we can recognize that a response we keep having is connected to a memory from our past. There is no need to spend a lot of time and effort trying to figure out exactly why we keep having a particular response—what matters is that we recognize that this response is so familiar and consistent, across very different contexts, that it's likely to be at least in part from something in our past rather than a response to what's happening now. That awareness can help us have compassion for ourselves and for the pain we're experiencing and can also help us clarify our feelings in the moment.

Mindfulness of Emotions and Physical Sensations

Now that we've explored some of the reasons our emotions can be muddy, let's try another mindfulness practice and see how it affects our muddy emotions. This is a challenging practice, so try not to expect too much from it this first time. If you haven't been practicing mindfulness regularly yet, you may find that you don't notice anything new about your emotions as you try this practice today. It can still be useful to get a sense of what it's like to bring awareness to these kinds of jumbled emotions, though.

For this practice, think of a time in the past week when your emotions were muddy. This might be a time when you felt generally distressed and agitated, or irritated and on edge, or easily reactive to small things that went wrong, or confused about how you were feeling. See if you can remember a time when you felt that your emotional responses did not match what was happening in the moment or you had no idea what you were feeling or why you were upset. If possible, choose something that remains unresolved, so that you still have reactions to it when you think about it.

First, write a brief description of the situation you have chosen in your notebook so that you can begin to get a clear memory of it.

Now think about the sensory experiences during this memory. What did you hear, see, smell, and feel during this event? What did you notice in your body? If you can't get a clear sense of the details of memory, just focus on the feeling that you remember and what that feels like in your body. Take a few minutes to explore the memory before you do the exercise.

Now download the audio recording of this exercise at the book website or read over the following guidelines for the practice below and then close the book and try the practice on your own for 5 to 10 minutes.

Begin by noticing the way you are sitting. Noticing where your body touches the chair or floor. Then gently bringing your awareness to your breath. Noticing where you feel it in your body. Noticing the sensations as you inhale and exhale. You may feel the breath in your belly, your chest, the back of your throat, or your nostrils. Just allowing your awareness to settle there for a moment as you feel yourself breathe.

As your awareness settles on this moment, allow your memory of this time you felt muddy emotions to arise. Picture yourself in the situation, noticing what you can see, the sounds you hear. [Pause for a minute.]

Then bring awareness to feelings in your body, noticing any tightness in your body. Seeing where you can feel the muddiness. You may notice your chest is tight, or your shoulders are hunched, or you have a pit in your stomach. Just noticing whatever sensations you have in your body during this time of muddy emotions.

As you continue to breathe into your body, remembering this time, noticing the physical sensations in your body, you may also notice thoughts running through your mind. As each thought arises, noticing it and then gently bringing your awareness back to the sensations in your body.

Just continue paying attention to any sensations in your body during this situation, as well as the emotions that arise. You may notice many emotions, or only a general state of distress. You may observe that the sensations in your body are connected to an emotional state. Whatever you notice, just allowing all of these experiences to unfold.

Noticing any urges to respond to your experience, and any desire to avoid your feelings.

Just continue paying attention to your experience, bringing curiousness and compassion to what you are experiencing. Observing what happens to you when you are feeling muddy emotions, without altering it or judging your experience. Noticing the way muddy emotions feel in your body.

Noticing any time you are trying to alter or judging your experience and just letting go, refocusing on the experience and the sensations in your body.

Noticing any efforts to push feelings away or efforts to hold on to feelings. Seeing how those efforts affect your breath and the sensations in your body. And continuing to breathe and allowing your experience to unfold while you remember this situation.

Observing how your feelings change or ways they don't change.

When your timer goes off, letting the memory go and bringing your awareness again to your breath and the present moment before you open your eyes.

After you practice this exercise, take a few moments to write down what you noticed in your notebook.

As we mentioned earlier, this can be a challenging exercise, so you may have noticed that challenge and wondered what else you were getting out of it. It can be helpful to practice the skills of mindfulness in states of distress or discomfort so that you'll be able to use these skills during the times you need them most—when feeling upset. In addition, sometimes practicing mindfulness can reduce reactivity, so that your emotions become slightly less muddy or overwhelming.

You may have had a moment in this exercise when you felt slightly less entangled in your responses, or you felt able to see your experience with a little bit more distance or perspective. You may have noticed thoughts or judgments that you had not realized you were having at the time. Or you may have realized a sense of sadness, loss, or fear that you were unaware of in the situation. Or you may have noticed how your responses were connected to something that happened in the past or that you fear may happen in the future. Any of these experiences gave you a brief taste of how mindfulness practice can change our relationship to our internal experiences and help us engage more directly in our lives. We'll continue with these practices so that you can have more moments like this (or your first moments like this) and discover how mindfulness may help you.

Reactions to Our Reactions

During the last mindfulness exercise, you may have noticed thoughts like "I'm being too emotional" or "I shouldn't get so worked up about these things." These critical and judgmental reactions to our emotional responses are part of being human but also commonly cause our emotions to become muddy. In fact, research has shown that experiencing worry or feelings of arousal does not necessarily lead to anxiety disorders. Anxiety disorders are associated with having negative or catastrophic responses to these feelings of anxiety and worry. Many people have worries, but people who worry excessively, in ways that interfere with their lives, have learned to worry about worrying and about the potential negative effects of their worry. Many people experience increases in their heart rate or shortness of breath but do not go on to develop panic disorder. Those who do have learned to respond to these signs of arousal with fear and worry, which increases their anxiety and worsens the arousal, starting a cycle of anxious responding that can be hard to stop. Research shows that people can also respond to experiences of anger, sadness, and even happiness with distress and that these reactions are associated with psychological symptoms.

> *Research has shown that it's not feeling worry that causes anxiety disorders but having negative responses to these feelings.*

Of course, no one has these reactions on purpose. We learn to respond negatively to our emotions, sensations, or thoughts in a number of different ways:

- When a really distressing event occurs, our responses at the time can become reminders of that event without our conscious awareness of the connection.
- A negative response from parents or other family members may teach us that our distress is dangerous and should be avoided.
- We may get praise for seeming "calm, cool, and collected" and criticism for being emotional, making us wish we were more calm and judging ourselves negatively when we're not.
- We may notice that other people *seem* to be less emotionally reactive than we are, and that may lead us to feel bad about our own responses. Of course, judging our internal states by other people's external states can blind us to the fact that they may be experiencing distress and worry as well; we just may not be able to observe their internal distress.

Mindfulness can help us notice these reactions to our reactions, and we can also learn, through this particular type of awareness, how to bring compassion to our experiences, no matter how many judgments automatically arise. This often takes a great deal of practice, because we have become so used to criticizing and judging our responses. Many people find that when they first try to cultivate this practice, they notice their judgments and judge them—which only intensifies the muddiness! With patience and practice, we can learn to bring compassion to our experiences and our judgments, no matter where in the cycle we are able to notice them.

Sometimes it can help to think of this practice as adding something to our awareness, rather than trying to take anything away. So when we have judgments or negative reactions, we don't have to try to get rid of those reactions, but we can add a sense of compassion and care for ourselves. When we see our responses as natural and human, it can be easier to continue to act in ways that matter to us, regardless of our emotional responses.

> Ramon felt a pit in his stomach and tapped his foot restlessly while he waited for Jack to come into his office for his performance review. He thought about the critical feedback he had to give and began to worry about how Jack would respond when he heard it. He noticed the signs of his anxiety and told himself to pull himself together and prepare to do his job. He had thoughts about how he was too sensitive and too emotional and that maybe he wasn't cut out to be a supervisor. Each time he noticed his anxiety, he worried that he would not be able to communicate clearly, and his anxiety continued to rise. His breathing was getting shallow and rapid, and he worried he would have a panic attack.
>
> Noticing the change in his breath reminded him of the book he was reading about mindfulness. He brought his attention to his breathing, noticing his inhalations and exhalations. He remembered reading that anxiety is a natural response in social situations and when we do things that are important to us. He reminded himself that this was his first time providing negative feedback in this new supervisory position, so his anxiety really was natural and understandable. He continued to feel uneasy, with an increase in anxiety when Jack walked into the room. Ramon focused on his intentions in providing this feedback to Jack, while feeling compassion for both Jack and himself in this challenging situation. He initially stumbled over his words, and was able to notice that that was a natural consequence of his anxiety. He took a breath and continued to provide clear feedback to Jack, while looking him in the eyes. Although Jack was clearly upset by the feedback, he told Ramon that he appreciated the clear communication and that he would try to follow his advice for ways to improve his performance.

Entangled, Hooked, Fused Relationship with Emotions

In the example above, Ramon was reactive to his anxious responses so that his responses began to get muddier. In addition, he began to see his response as defining him (he is "too sensitive" or "too emotional"). This kind of fusion with our emotional experiences can further muddy and intensify our responses. If you see yourself as an anxious person and you see anxiety as bad, it is no wonder that you have a negative reaction to any indicator of anxiety. Yet these reactions can make you feel your emotions even more intensely and also make it even more difficult to fully understand the complexity of your emotional response.

So reactivity to emotions leads us to be more entangled and fused with our emotional experiences, while being entangled with these experiences makes us more reactive, so that the cycle continues to escalate into even more muddy emotional responses. Another way of thinking about this is that we get "hooked" or entangled so that we feel all wrapped up in the emotions we are having, instead of seeing these emotions as rising and falling over the course of our lives. And again, reactivity to the emotions gets us more hooked so that our emotional experience does in fact seem to settle on us and not change very easily.

> *Reactivity and entanglement with emotional experiences perpetuates a cycle of muddied emotions.*

Again, mindful awareness can help us disentangle from our responses and get unhooked. You may have noticed in the preceding exercise that you had a moment of seeing your emotional response rise and fall, or seeing some variability in your emotion. You may find when you're doing your mindfulness practice that you notice a feeling and that you experience it as arising, rather than experiencing it as defining you. This experience of the ebb and flow of emotions helps us put a little bit of space between ourselves and our emotional responses, which can reduce the muddiness of these responses.

Sometimes people talk about mindfulness as though the goal were to *detach* from emotional experiences or be unaffected by them. But there is an important difference between being able to observe our emotions, and feel some space between us and them, and being numb to them or detached from them all together. These are still our emotional responses and, as we discussed in the last chapter, they provide important information to us. So the goal is not to buffer ourselves from them or denounce them in any way. In fact, as we discuss in the next chapter, trying to get away from our emotions is another way that we can get more entangled in them and that they can become even muddier.

EXERCISE **Noticing clear and muddy emotions**

To begin to bring more awareness to how your emotions can become muddy, continue monitoring your emotional responses this week, and note whether the responses seem to be muddy or clear. You may want to follow Dex (from the beginning of Chapter 6) or Ramon's examples and take a moment to breathe and see whether you can observe some clear emotions in the midst of muddy reactions. Jot down the emotions you notice and whether they seem to be muddy or clear. See what you can learn about your own emotional responses by doing this exercise.

8

the allure and cost
of trying to control your
internal experience

If fear, anxiety, sadness, and other emotions are natural human responses, why have we come to respond to them as dangerous, negative, painful, and problematic? Societal and cultural forces, along with our personal learning histories and beliefs, shape how we view and respond to emotions. As we discussed in the last chapter, our critical judgments and reactions muddy our emotions, increasing their frequency and intensity and making them seem even more complicated, frightening, and undesirable. In this chapter, we explore more deeply our automatic and habitual responses to anxiety and other emotions, particularly the instinct we all have to try to control these responses. As you'll see, the very steps we take to try to cope with anxiety add to its power over our lives. Fortunately, though, we can bring flexibility and choice back into our lives by developing a mindful awareness of the tendency to try to control our emotions and by cultivating a more accepting, compassionate, and mindful stance toward anxiety.

Humans are faced with a challenging paradox. Our prime directive seems to be to create and live a full and meaningful life. We're often guided by the philosophy that we should seek opportunities to experience pleasure, enjoyment, and satisfaction and avoid encounters that could bring pain and suffering. Unfortunately, living a fulfilling life involves putting ourselves in situations that inevitably stir up painful thoughts and feelings. How do we foster a deep connection with a friend while shielding ourselves from the pain and sadness of missing her when she is gone? Doesn't taking risks such as moving to another part of the country, accepting a job opportunity, or going back to school bring nervous anticipation as well as excitement? To become an accomplished musician, wouldn't you have to risk feeling frustrated, bored, or even incompetent as you practice the skills and exercises that may also eventually bring satisfaction and pride? It's a universal paradox that the potential for emotional pain seems inherent in every activity or situation that we might pursue. How do we resolve this paradox? In this chapter we explore three possible options: playing it safe, taking control, or taking a mindful accepting stance toward anxiety (and other sources of emotional pain).

Before reading on, take a few moments to reflect on whether you have ever felt stuck in this paradox. How have you tried to resolve it for your own life?

Common Responses Aimed at Resolving the Paradox

- Play it safe by carefully choosing a path in life that you hope will protect you from anxiety and other forms of emotional pain.
- Focus all your efforts on controlling anxiety in the hope that once you are anxiety-free you can pursue the things that matter most to you.
- Develop an accepting and mindful stance toward emotions and be willing to experience the full range of emotions that arise when you fully participate in life.

Option 1: Playing It Safe

Paula grew up in a chaotic but lonely home. The daughter of an introverted and alcoholic mother and a meek and often absent father, her physical and emotional needs were frequently neglected. At a very young age Paula became self-sufficient; she survived on cold cereal for supper until she could reach the stovetop to fix hot meals like macaroni and cheese or hot dogs. The family did not own their own washing machine, but Paula made sure to rinse out her clothes in the bathroom sink each night so they would be clean for school. Paula faced many childhood struggles alone. Although there were kindly and caring teachers, neighbors, and even relatives who would have intervened had they known the extent of Paula's neglect, she lived in fear of being removed from the only home and family she knew. By all appearances, Paula was a well-behaved child and a good student who never caused any trouble at school. But underneath her quiet, unassuming exterior, she was a lonely, scared child.

Despite her difficult childhood, Paula has built a relatively secure and stable life for herself. She is a hard worker and has been employed with the same company for the past 15 years. Although Paula gets along well with her coworkers, has a few acquaintances she sometimes sees a movie with on weekends, and occasionally goes on dates, she doesn't feel particularly close to anyone. Paula struggles with social anxiety; she is afraid if people get to know her well they will view her as damaged and flawed and reject her. Still, she holds out hope that someday she will find a partner she can trust and confide in. Once she meets someone who demonstrates his trustworthiness and she is certain she will not be judged or let down, she will allow herself to have an open, intimate relationship. But for now, she will continue to keep a safe distance between herself and others. Hasn't she been hurt enough in her life?

Many of us attempt to resolve the paradox by making choices about relationships, jobs, opportunities, and pastimes that limit our potential contact with pain, disappointment, sadness, and worry. We may not completely give up on the possibility of a fuller life, but we make compromises and restrict options in an attempt to play it safe. Most of us would agree that Paula has every reason to be self-protective. She had a terribly difficult childhood and doesn't deserve to be hurt anymore.

Unfortunately, although this seems like a reasonable and logical option, upon closer examination it becomes clear that this attempt to resolve the paradox is fatally flawed. Regardless of how careful we are it's impossible to avoid fear, sadness, and anger. As we discussed in Chapter 6, these emotions are part of our basic biological programming. They focus our attention, communicate the significance of an event, and ready us for action. No matter how hard we try to protect ourselves, we will inevitably come into contact with loss and emotional pain in our lives.

Remember that in addition to being hard wired to avoid pain, we are compelled to seek relationships and challenges in our life. Paula may fear the pain of disappointment, grief, or humiliation that she pictures will follow rejection, but like all humans, she has an innate desire to be part of a social network. Keeping a "safe" distance from others may protect her from the pain associated specifically with rejection, but doing so will undoubtedly elicit feelings of sadness, loneliness, and fear. Ironically, in her attempt to shield herself from pain, Paula will create a life that will naturally elicit it.

Part of the reason that many of us, including Paula, get stuck trying to solve the paradox by playing it safe is that *our belief that certain rules for living should work is stronger than our ability to objectively review the evidence in our own lives.* For example, the idea that building up walls protects one from pain is pretty common in our society. Mindfulness can help us more accurately reflect on whether this strategy could ever be successful for anyone. Beginner's mind (a

> *The fatal flaw in playing it safe becomes clear when you take a close, hard look at the evidence for its efficacy.*

mindfulness skill introduced in Chapter 5) can help us observe both the efficacy and the consequences of playing it safe, rather than just taking its usefulness as a given. This can help us stop habitually blaming ourselves and attributing the failure of the "playing it safe" plan to our own weaknesses and shortcomings and see instead that the plan itself is flawed. Mindfulness can help us observe the full range of emotions we experience when we limit our lives to avoid pain, even if some of our responses are automatic and typically outside of our awareness.

EXERCISE **Are there times you have played it safe?**

Paula had some very dramatic reasons to develop the habit of "playing it safe." But many of us, even if we don't have the childhood experiences Paula did, learn to try to protect ourselves from emotional pain by avoiding situations where we might be hurt or disappointed. Reflect on some of the choices you have made to "play it safe." Are there relationships you have avoided or kept at bay? Job or career opportunities you have passed up? Have those choices brought you peace, calmness, and well-being, or is anxiety still present in your life? Have the choices brought additional emotional pain—disappointment, sadness, anger ... or negative thoughts about yourself?

Option 2: Take Control of Anxiety and Other Painful Reactions

Louis's mother had lived with severe panic disorder her whole life. Her struggle weighed heavily on the family, and Louis's father coped by spending increasingly longer days, nights, and weekends at the office. As a result, much of the household burden fell to Louis, who was an only child. By the time he was a teenager, Louis's mom was no longer willing to leave the house and was relying on Louis to run all her weekly errands. Not only was he charged with the weekly grocery shopping, but he also purchased all of his mother's clothing and other personal items. Although these responsibilities left Louis with little time to participate in school activities or hang out with friends, he fulfilled them willingly. It pained him to see his mother struggle so intensely, and he was grateful for the opportunity to ease her suffering.

Although Louis, now an adult, is also prone to frequent panic attacks, he is determined to live his life differently from his mom. His goal is to live an engaged and meaningful life, and he doesn't intend to let panic hold him back. He wants to be in a committed relationship, achieve success as a restaurateur, travel, and volunteer in his community. Louis is firm in his belief that to live the life he wants he must gain control and mastery over his anxiety. He is active in several online dating services, faithfully reading the profile of at least five new men a week to increase the chances that he will find someone who has the potential to be his soulmate. In the past month he has set up dates with three men. Before each date, Louis goes for a long run, hoping to burn off his excessive anxiety. He always arrives at the appointed meeting site first so that he can quickly down a few glasses of wine to calm his nerves. If he notices himself beginning to get nervous, he excuses himself, heads to the men's room, and tries to pull himself together with a firm internal lecture on the dangers of ending up like his mom.

Despite his best efforts, Louis is finding it harder and harder to control his anxiety, and he is beginning to feel a bit hopeless. Sometimes using distraction techniques, self-talk, and a few glasses of wine really helps him manage his anxiety. But other times, no matter what he tries, the anxiety sneaks up on him. Louis is afraid he is losing the motivation and focus he needs to stay on top of his emotions. He wishes he could have the discipline and focus he had as a teen. What scares Louis most are his thoughts. He knows he must keep his confidence up to succeed, but nagging doubts and thoughts that he is weak and bound to fail are eating away at him.

EXERCISE **Advice on ways to control your anxiety**

People try all different methods to control their anxiety (and other emotions). Consider each of the following statements. Have you ever been given this advice as a way to manage your anxiety? Do you personally believe the statements to be true? Have you successfully incorporated any of these strategies into your own life?

- Distract yourself with thoughts about something else.
- Find something productive to do to get your mind off your anxiety.
- Try to think about your positive attributes.
- Don't be weak; give yourself a lecture about trying harder.
- Watch television.
- Have a drink (like a glass of wine or a beer) or a cigarette to calm your nerves.
- Take a sleeping pill or some other prescribed or over-the-counter medication to help you get some rest.

- Eat some ice cream, chips, or other junk food.
- Engage in retail therapy (in other words, go shopping).
- Ask other people for reassurance.
- Carry something around with you that makes you feel a little safer.
- Exercise.
- Find someone to talk to or hang out with.

Chances are, if you picked up this book, you care deeply about living a full and satisfying life. Many of us, like Louis, believe that controlling our anxiety is the first step toward a better life. If fears and doubts creep in, we think, they need to be replaced swiftly with self-confidence and a positive outlook. Many of us invest considerable time and energy into these control efforts. Yet they often meet with little success, which can leave us feeling ineffective, stuck, and even a little hopeless.

Why, then, do so many of us struggle with controlling our anxious thoughts and emotions? Two major assumptions underlie the belief that controlling anxiety and quelling negative thoughts are the first steps to leading a more fulfilling life.

Assumption 1: Humans Can Control Anxiety (and Other Emotional Responses)

Many of us believe that control over anxiety is possible—that others have done it even if we have not. We assume we haven't been able to achieve this control because we have some personality flaw or we're just not motivated. Interestingly, research suggests that once we experience a particular emotion or thought, we cannot simply change what we think or feel through sheer will or determination.

If you have ever had trouble falling asleep, you can probably relate to the phenomenon that trying to suppress a thought or emotion can exacerbate it. Imagine you're lying in bed, trying to get to sleep because you know you have a big day ahead of you. You feel anxious and jittery, but you would like to suppress those emotions and instead feel calm

> *There is evidence that trying to suppress a painful emotion or challenging thought can actually make it occur more frequently, last longer, and cause more distress.*

and relaxed. You toss and turn, and when you glance at the clock and see that it's approaching midnight, you really start to worry. "What if I can't get to sleep? I'll be exhausted tomorrow. I can't function if I don't get enough sleep." Have you ever noticed that the harder you try to fall asleep, the more your efforts backfire? The higher the stakes, the more impossible it is to control your sleep?

The same kind of thing can happen when we try to control anxiety. Imagine if you were hooked up to an extremely sensitive machine that could recognize with 100% accuracy whether you were feeling anxious. The slightest worry, the fluttering of an increasing heart rate, even subtle changes in body temperature would be detected easily by this device. Imagine that your job was simply to stay completely calm and relaxed while attached to this sophisticated piece of equipment. Using all the control strategies at your disposal—distraction, positive imagery, self-criticism, motivation to overcome your anxiety—would you be able to maintain a state of calm if you were told that becoming anxious would cause the machine to explode—and, of course, that if the machine exploded, you were likely to be seriously injured? It would be virtually impossible to stay completely calm and relaxed in this environment. Why? *Because, as we have discussed throughout the book, humans are hardwired to feel anxious when in a threatening situation. No amount of self-control and determination can override that natural response.*

In contrast, we could exert some control over our behavior in this situation. For example, someone might decide to decline the offer to be hooked up to the machine. Another might be up for the challenge and choose to maintain a stoic exterior while being pummeled by exploding machine parts.

> *It's impossible to stop a natural emotional response like anxiety from occurring by sheer will.*

We often can exert control over the choices we make about how to behave in different situations, but it is impossible to stop a natural emotional response like anxiety from occurring by sheer will.

Interestingly, this inability to control emotions, particularly fear, is actually evolutionarily adaptive. It makes sense that the part of our brain that responds to threat does so quickly and automatically, without any involvement from the parts of our brain involved in planning or integrating information. This allows us to respond to any potential threat without deliberation. It also makes sense that the parts of our brain that regulate our emotions respond more slowly, with less rapid connections between them and the parts of our brain that generate emotion. Determining safety is much less vital than determining risk, particularly in places filled with physical and social dangers, so a brain that will respond quickly to threat and be slower to recover will optimize survival. Unfortunately, such a brain does not optimize emotional comfort, leading to the frustrations inherent in trying to control these emotional responses.

Trying to get rid of the difficult or painful ones is not the only way we try to control our emotions. We also sometimes try to hold on to or re-create the emotions we find desirable. Take Veronica, a single woman who is actively seeking a life partner. Recently she has been spending a lot of time with two particular men, Billy and Don. Billy is handsome, athletic, considerate, and easygoing. He is a pediatric oncologist at the local hospital and spends his free time hiking and bicycling, trying new restaurants, and volunteering at a homeless shelter. Veronica loves spending time with Billy. She appreciates his thoughtfulness and enjoys his dry sense of humor. Last month, Billy accompanied Veronica to her cousin's wedding. Now every time Veronica talks to her friends and family they comment on what a great guy Billy is. Although Veronica knows that Billy would make a wonderful partner, she just doesn't feel a romantic spark.

In contrast, Veronica is extremely attracted to Don. He is attractive and charismatic, always the center of attention. Veronica loves Don's romantic side; he can be so sweet, funny, and engaging when he calls to wish her good night. Unfortunately, Veronica never knows when he will actually call. Sometimes he calls every night for a week, and other times a month will pass with no contact. To his credit, Don is completely honest and up front: he warned Veronica that he had no interest in pursuing a committed relationship. She told herself it would be fun just to date him for a while, no strings attached. Unfortunately, her heart had a plan of its own.

If Veronica had control over her emotions, she would absolutely make herself fall in love with Billy and out of love with Don. But just as it's impossible to push away fear and anxiety, we can't switch feelings of love on and off. Once again, however, Veronica can exert control over her behavior. She can choose to break off the relationship with Don, although doing so will not prevent her from feeling sad, lonely, and disappointed, at least in the short term.

Sometimes we engage in a subtle, complex control strategy aimed at keeping our current positive emotions in check to avoid the risk of future negative emotions. Jemeka, for example, was initially very excited about a new job prospect but quickly backed off to avoid potential hurt. "The hours, location, and pay are perfect," Jemeka excitedly told her friend Maria about the newly posted job available in the library of her son's elementary school. "Exactly what I've been looking for to get my life back on track!" But then Maria warned, "Don't go getting your hopes up too high." Like most friends, Maria had seen Jemeka through many tearful disappointments, and she wanted to shield her friend from additional pain. Jemeka immediately pictured how she would feel if she didn't get the job and quickly assured her friend, "Oh, don't worry. I'm not expecting anything at all. I mean, there might be a lot of other people applying, and I'm sure lots of them will be more qualified than I am." With her friend as witness, Jemeka put on a dispassionate face, but privately after applying for the job she vacillated every day between fervently hoping she'd get the job and harshly criticizing herself for doing so.

On the surface, it seems to makes sense that the best method for preventing future disappointment would be to suppress excitement and hope. Unfortunately, hope and excitement are the emotions that propel us to take chances, to apply for a job, ask someone on a date, or audition for a part. Disappointment is a natural indicator that we wanted something and didn't get it. No matter how much we try to rationalize ourselves out of having those feelings, there is no way to take chances without them.

Trying to control anxiety not only reveals that troubling emotions are unavoidable; sometimes it also leads us to create self-fulfilling prophecies. For example, Anwah had a history of painful breakups, and she was determined to prevent herself from getting hurt again. So when she met Lata, even though she felt a strong physical and emotional connection, Anwah decided to "play it cool." She repeatedly canceled dates and purposely ignored Lata's texts to keep some distance between them and minimize any loss she might eventually feel over a breakup. Although Anwah exerted significant control over her behavior by turning down some of Lata's requests, privately she felt her attraction to Lata growing. The fact that she couldn't make those feelings evaporate on command frightened her even more; the more intense her attraction, the more devastating a breakup seemed likely to be. So she acted more and more disinterested in Lata. Ultimately Anwah was so successful in hiding her true feelings that Lata decided to pursue a relationship with someone else. Despite the stoic appearance that she maintained, Anwah *was* in fact devastated by the loss.

Assumption 2: Anxiety and Negative Thoughts Prevent Us from Living Fulfilling Lives

Many people try to control their emotions because they think they need to sweep them out of the way before pursuing the relationships, challenges, and activities that contribute to a fulfilling life. Remember Selena, the teacher introduced in Chapter 2 who took a job for which she was overqualified, planning to eliminate her fear of public speaking before she went back to the work she loved? Selena had put her life on hold to embark on a private journey of self-improvement. On the surface, this "tune-up" approach seems reasonable. Drain all the anxiety from the system, crank up the self-confidence, replace all those old worried thoughts with positive thinking, and go for a "practice" test drive before taking a risk on the highway of life.

Unfortunately, mindfully observing and specifically bringing beginner's mind to evaluate the true effectiveness of this approach, often yields new insight. As Selena discovered, putting one's life on hold or restricting opportunities during a self-improvement stage naturally elicits some pretty painful emotions, such as boredom and sadness. And although it seems like one could conjure up positive thoughts and self-confidence through self-reflection, these reactions are much more likely to emerge from interaction and engagement. Socializing with a friend, venturing out into a new environment, and taking on a risky challenge are far more likely to elicit joy, happiness, contentment, excitement, pride, and confidence than engaging in internal debate or even a marathon of self-help book reading.

Furthermore, although most of us are inclined to feel first and act later, we are not required to respond that way. You don't have to feel particularly energized before taking a run around the lake. Paradoxically, you're more likely to feel revived *after* exercising. Similarly, the authors of a book don't need to feel enthused and inspired before each writing session. In fact, the act of writing is what typically elicits those responses. Most important, you do not have to feel confident and worry-free before trying something new, taking a risk, or accepting a challenge.

Ironically, taking these actions is what's most likely to boost confidence. You do not need to be fearless to live; you need only be courageous. As Ambrose Redmoon wrote, "Courage is not the absence of fear, but rather the judgment that something else is more important than fear."

If Control Is Not a Reasonable Option, Why Are We So Attached to It?

If you take a step back and think about it, it's sort of strange how persistent we are about trying to control our anxiety when our own experience tells us it isn't working. Usually humans learn pretty quickly from experience. A toddler who thinks the pretty, shiny radiator would be fun to touch quickly learns it is hot and she should stay away. The teenager who tries a shortcut home from school only to find that the hilly terrain makes his walk longer and more arduous will quickly find an alternate route. One case of food poisoning is all it takes to develop an aversion to sushi. So why do we keep trying to control our anxiety when our efforts repeatedly fail? Why do researchers who study control and write books on the topic persist in occasionally attempting to control their fears and disappointments?

The message is ingrained in us by society.

One cultural message that pervades American society is that it is valuable and desirable to use logic and reason to manage emotion. Being in control of one's emotions is often equated with positive qualities such as competence, balance, and achievement.

Take a moment and notice the thoughts and judgments that come to mind when hearing someone described in the following way: "She is such an emotional person." Would you consider this a compliment? Despite the fact that emotions are universal and helpful, we're often exposed to cultural messages that certain emotional responses are undesirable, a sign of weakness or character defects. We often get the message from those around us that emotions like anxiety prevent us from achieving our goals and living a fulfilling and meaningful life.

Even at a very young age, children are given both subtle and obvious messages that they should control their emotions. It's perfectly natural for children starting kindergarten to feel some apprehension and fear. Children may also feel sad about the transition and miss spending time with their parents or caregivers. A parent might respond to her child's reaction with validation and additional information: "I can understand why you feel a little scared. It's a new situation and you don't know what to expect. A lot of kids feel this way. Your teacher actually expects that everyone will feel a little scared, and she has lots of fun activities planned to make it a little easier to get used to being at school. I will be back to pick you up in 2 hours, and you can tell me all about your day." On the other hand, another parent might attempt to reassure her child (and herself) by saying "Oh, stop it! You're not scared, are you? Don't feel that way; everything will be fine. You're not a baby anymore." Although this second parent may be trying to be helpful, a child who is feeling afraid is likely to feel confused or invalidated by this message. He or she may interpret that message to mean that (1) feeling afraid in this situation is wrong or bad in some way and (2) I should be able to get rid of or change my emotional state. And if a child repeatedly receives the message that certain emotions are undesirable and should be avoided, particularly from parents or other adults in a position of authority, these messages are likely to be internalized and personalized.

Even as adults, we frequently respond to others' painful emotions with logic and reason in an attempt to change their feelings. We try to convince the disappointed job candidate that her dream position would have really been a dead-end job. We aim to soothe the grieving widower by stressing how his partner is now at peace. We present a list of evidence to our worried friend as to why she has no cause for fear. We justify and defend our position to those we anger. On the surface these responses may seem reasonable and helpful. Yet when we are on the receiving end of the message, often we don't find the advice tremendously helpful. We are hardwired to feel emotions in response to events. Losses bring disappointment and sadness. Risk and uncertainty bring worry and fear. When we are wronged, we feel angry. And although these emotions do fade in intensity with time and new experiences, it is important to acknowledge and accept their appearance.

EXERCISE **Your history with emotion and control efforts**

Spend a few minutes reflecting on your thoughts about emotions and their expression. How did your caregivers deal with their emotions or respond to yours? Do you remember people telling you to control or suppress your emotions? Can you think of models you had for expressing emotions or models for suppressing or controlling them? What kinds of experiences have you had that might affect your motivation to try to control your emotional responses?

Others seem to be able to control their emotional responses.

Because we are not privy to others' personal experiences, we don't always see their private struggles with difficult and painful emotions. In fact, we often judge our insides, which we know intimately, by other people's outsides, because that is all we can see. Often we are surprised and taken aback to find a coworker is struggling with suicidal thoughts, a neighbor has a drinking problem, or the lovely couple down the road engages in domestic violence. When you ride with people on the elevator or exchange pleasantries in the line at the grocery store, they may appear calm and in control. Outward appearances do not always reflect the struggles within.

As children, we are most at risk for imagining that the grown-ups around us are in control of their inner experiences. Most young children express their emotions quite strongly—crying when sad or angry or clutching for help when afraid. In contrast, most adults keep the expression of their emotional experiences private, so children can come to believe that it is desirable and grown-up to feel things less strongly.

Ironically, sometimes a parent will demand that a child change his emotional response because the parent himself is struggling with emotions. For example, George and his 5-year-old son Tommy recently spent the day together at an amusement park. The blistering hot weather didn't discourage crowds of visitors from flocking to the park. As the afternoon wore on, George felt himself grow more and more irritated by the long lines, screaming children, and scorching sun. He kept trying to suppress his feelings and push on, but it wasn't working, and he knew he needed a break from the park. "One last ride," George warned as Tommy eagerly led him to the spinning teacups, which was not only Tommy's favorite ride, but apparently one of the most popular in the park. Forty-five minutes later they finally reached the front of the line, only to learn that the ride would be closed temporarily for maintenance.

The indifferent manner of the ride operator as Tommy burst into tears just added fuel to an already flaming fire. George felt overwhelmed by his emotions and lashed out at his son. "How dare you cry after everything I did for you today? I bought you souvenirs and snacks, took you on every single ride, and now you are acting like a baby. Grow up and pull yourself together," George hissed into his son's ear as he pulled him by the arm toward the parking lot.

Clearly, George was struggling with his own emotions. He found his own sadness, disappointment, and anger too much to manage, and seeing his son upset only made those emotions grow in intensity. In a desperate attempt to escape those painful emotions, George focused his effort on trying to get his son to feel differently and to stop crying. In other words, because Tommy's pain was contributing to George's distress, and George couldn't control his own emotional state, he demanded that his son control his. Unfortunately, from Tommy's perspective, the message from his dad was that emotions can be controlled and you are bad and flawed if you cannot suppress your feelings.

Control works so well in other domains.

Let's say you wanted to build a patio in your backyard. You might start by creating a plan, removing the overgrown brush and hauling away rocks to clear the space, shopping around for pavers, and so forth. There is a series of concrete, controllable steps you can take to get the patio done. If you wanted to prepare a special dinner, you could search for recipes, create a grocery list, shop for the necessary ingredients, and then cook. Many of the problems we encounter in our daily life can be tackled through planning, persistence, and hard work. Many of the goals we aspire to achieve can be broken down into concrete steps to be completed. Unfortunately, internal states are not as responsive to this problem-solving approach.

Sometimes we **can** control or suppress our feelings.

Alex gets pretty nervous in social situations, and she finds that a few glasses of white wine can put her at ease and help her make small talk. Latesha has a needle phobia, but her mom can test her blood sugar if Latesha is engrossed in her favorite television show. Jessica struggles with performance anxiety before skating competitions, but she has a pre-event ritual of listening to her favorite song and warming up with her lucky gloves that helps to calm her nerves. Stewart finds that a few minutes of deep breathing before a staff meeting quiets the panicky feelings that might otherwise interfere with his ability to present his report. Alberto, racked with worry as he awaits the results of his daughter Luisa's bone marrow test, plans a large family dinner the night before the medical appointment to distract him from his concerns.

Although both scientific research and personal experience suggest that attempting to control or suppress anxiety often results in a rebound effect of more distress and interference, there are absolutely times in which we are able to successfully push bothersome anxious thoughts and feelings away. At least for a short time, distraction techniques, rituals, alcohol or drug use, and other strategies can reduce our anxiety. These short-term successes with control often leave us believing that if we just tried harder or focused more we could gain mastery and control over our anxiety *all* the time. Research with both animals and humans has shown that the best way to ensure a behavior occurs over and over again is to reward it only occasionally. If a dog gets a treat each time he performs a new trick, over time he may demonstrate the trick less frequently. But if the owner randomly rewards the trick, the dog's behavior will persist. Similarly, because control strategies work in reducing anxiety every so often, we are much more likely to keep on trying them.

> *The fact that control strategies do occasionally reduce anxiety makes us keep trying them.*

Unfortunately, even though control over anxiety is sometimes possible, the strategies are not always readily available or reliable, and there is no guarantee that they will work at the crucial moment. When Alex has to attend work luncheons, she is extremely uncomfortable because no alcohol is available and yet she is still expected to socialize with her coworkers and clients. Similarly, Latesha is panic-stricken when she has to undergo a medical procedure that involves a needle stick in the doctor's office, where no television is available to distract her. When Jessica's pre-competition ritual didn't calm her nerves before regionals, she felt so helpless and out of control that she withdrew from the event. Similarly, Stewart was devastated when his preparatory breathing strategy failed him before a significant meeting at corporate headquarters. In addition to being anxious, he was distracted throughout the meeting by an internal tirade of criticism over not being able to control anxiety and worry about how he would endure these meetings in the future.

Control efforts are also flawed in that they do not seem to yield any long-term reduction in anxiety. The fears, worries, and butterflies in the stomach always return, often with more intensity and frequency. Repeatedly using control-directed strategies (with some successes and some failures) can also bring its own negative consequences. Although it's unlikely that breathing or visiting with family could result in long-term negative consequences, other control strategies such as overeating or alcohol and drug misuse can become extremely problematic. Engaging in these strategies can also lead us to become more and more consumed with shoring up and improving our efforts, which distracts our attention and energy from other, more meaningful activities.

Finally, these strategies often set off a cycle that entangles us in muddied emotions. For instance, if a psychologist is asked to give a talk in front of a large audience, fear might be a clear emotional response to being asked to do something that could result in social evaluation. If she then judges this fear negatively and takes it as a sign that she is a failure, a fraud, etc., she is likely to start to feel other muddy emotions such as shame and guilt. So, in that moment, she has a very complex and intense emotional response that includes both clear and muddy emotions. In response to that very intense emotional response, she might try unsuccessfully to control her reactions. If control backfires, she is likely to be left with a complex array of muddy emotions fueled by her self-blame and disgust over not being able to exert control. This reaction is likely to cue ever stronger control efforts. This cycle of feeling a clear emotion, judging it, attempting to control it, feeling more intensely, judging more intensely, and trying harder to control can lead to significant distress. The more intense this cycle gets, the muddier our emotions get. At this point, then, these emotions don't provide us with the useful information that clearer emotions do. They're so jumbled up that it is hard to know what they are telling us anymore.

Anxiety is most commonly a muddy emotion. It often contains within it clear responses of fear in response to the present situation, along with muddier responses to what we tell ourselves the situation represents, and more muddy responses that come from trying not to be so anxious. It is quite reasonable to want to control anxiety, since intense anxiety can interfere with our ability to do things. For instance, if we feel afraid before we take a test, we're likely to want to stop feeling this way, because we think fear may make it harder to remember things on the test. In actuality, fear in this situation is communicating to us that the test matters in some way and the fear motivates us to study, show up on time, narrow our focus of attention on the test, and so on. However, if we believe that fear is a problem—that it means we're flawed, that it will interfere with our performance—we can become highly motivated to try not to feel afraid. Those efforts are likely to create an intense and muddy emotional reaction that will probably interfere with our performance on the test.

Option 3: Cultivating a Mindful Stance

Adopting an accepting, mindful stance toward thoughts, emotions, images, memories, and bodily sensations involves allowing fear, worry, and other troubling internal experiences to be present and diminishing the power they have as obstacles to valued living. As we'll discuss in the next chapter, acceptance should not be confused with surrender or resignation. We're not suggesting that you give up and resign yourself to the fact that you must live with unbearable levels of anxiety or worry. This option involves using mindfulness practice to develop a better awareness of clear emotions and to allow them to unfold and serve their natural function, minimize the presence and power of muddy emotions, and actively incorporate valued living into your daily life.

Much of the anxiety-related distress and life interference that people struggle with is driven by critical and controlling reactions to clear emotions that produce muddy emotions and prevent values-consistent behavior. Although the evidence suggests that it is impossible to consistently and permanently control or suppress clear emotions, you can exert some control in other ways that will make a difference in your life. First and foremost, you do have the ability to exert significant control over your behavior. Choosing to be the sort of parent, partner, and friend that you value, pursuing work or educational programs that matter to you or meet the needs of your family, and engaging in satisfying hobbies or community action events are all actions over which you can have considerable control. It is likely that your struggle to control anxiety and worry has pulled you away from taking action in these areas — maybe by taking up your attention, maybe by causing you to lose some faith in your ability to make changes and move ahead, maybe because you fear taking action and feeling even more anxiety. Mindfulness practice involves bringing a new stance toward your anxiety that reduces its interfering properties and allows you to engage more freely in these valued activities.

Choosing option 3 involves changing your focus a bit. Up to this point it's as if you've been involved in a time-consuming, draining, continuous tug-of-war with a monster. That monster represents your most private and personal fears and worries. Between you and the monster is a deep, dark, seemingly bottomless pit. Your primary focus of attention has been to overcome the monster in the tug-of-war, or at least hold your ground so that you are not dragged into the pit. You've been pulling with all your might, trying your best to overcome the monster, but the harder you pull, the harder the monster pulls on the other side, and it seems like you are edging closer and closer to the pit. You are not required to win this tug-of-war if you choose option 3. Instead, taking a mindful stance toward anxiety involves actually dropping the rope, letting go of the struggle, and turning toward what matters to you in your life. It's possible that you will continue to hear the monster scream, groan, and threaten you. But as long as you refuse to engage in a tug-of-war, as long as you're willing to let go of your struggle with anxiety, it will remain harmless. The choice of whether to struggle with anxiety or to let it be is in your control.

Letting it be involves not enduring unbearable anxiety but simply being *willing* to experience uncomfortable thoughts and feelings—clear emotions. Being willing does not mean subjecting yourself to

> *To struggle with anxiety or let it be? The choice is in your control.*

feeling constantly anxious or overwhelmed, or that the answer to your difficulties is just to brace yourself to feel the full and overwhelming tide of negative thoughts and feelings. Through mindfulness practice, the goal will be to change the relationship you have with your thoughts and feelings, to bring some curiosity and compassion to the responses you have, to learn to tune in to your emotions and understand how they pull you to respond in certain ways, and to bring some flexibility and choice to the actions you take.

EXERCISE **Noticing control efforts**

To help increase your awareness of your control efforts, try a new monitoring exercise for the next week or two. When you notice anxiety, worry, or any other painful emotion or thoughts arising, make an entry in your notebook. Note the date and situation and, using your mindfulness skills, tune in to the full range of thoughts and emotions you are experiencing. Next, pay attention to any urges you had to suppress, control, or otherwise change your experience. Make a note of any obvious or subtle ways you tried to control your responses. When you begin to pay attention to your control efforts, you may find that judgments or criticisms arise. Notice these and continue practicing kindness and compassion toward your experiences. Remember that urges to control painful thoughts and emotions are a natural, often overlearned human response. Becoming aware of your urges to control is a first step toward responding to anxiety with mindfulness.

9

acceptance and willingness

INCREASING FLEXIBILITY AND OPENING UP
TO NEW POSSIBILITIES

The Guest House

This being human is a guest house.
Every morning a new arrival.

A joy, a depression, a meanness,
Some momentary awareness comes
as an unexpected visitor.

Welcome and entertain them all!
Even if they're a crowd of sorrows,
who violently sweep your house
empty of its furniture,

still treat each guest honorably.
He may be clearing you out
for some new delight.

The dark thought, the shame, the malice.
meet them at the door laughing,
And invite them in.

Be grateful for whoever comes,
because each has been sent
as a guide from beyond.
    —RUMI *(translated by Barks & Moyne, 1995)*

People have a variety of responses when they first encounter "The Guest House." An extremely common response is "Why in the world would I ever graciously host a pack of sorrows, worries, and cruelties?" Many of us have barred our doors with padlocks and deadbolts, a chair jammed under the doorknob for good measure, in the hopes of keeping these shady characters away. Sometimes people sort of agree with the idea in theory but struggle to see how this approach will bring them relief from their struggles with anxiety. Still others readily accept the concept but are uncertain about how to incorporate it into their lives. Regardless of your initial reaction, we invite you to consider how you might come to treat anxiety and its associates as honorable guests in the service of a fuller and freer life. A number of mindfulness exercises introduced in the following pages are available to help.

What Exactly Does It Mean to Be Accepting and Willing?

Acceptance and willingness are strongly interrelated. *Acceptance* simply refers to letting go of the struggle against the reality of what "is" in a given moment. As a working parent, every so often, usually on a day during which a time-sensitive meeting is scheduled or some last piece of work is needed to meet a critical deadline, and when my husband is traveling out of town, the universe will present me (S. M. O.) with a vomiting child or a snowstorm severe enough to warrant a school closing in my suburb, but not strong enough to disrupt life in the city where I work. Inevitably, I go through a bit of a process before I am able to accept this reality: "No! This can't happen today of all days! It's not fair! Why couldn't I be on a work trip this week? If Sam would just wash his hands more frequently, maybe we could get through a month without a sick day!" I am not proud to admit it, but occasionally, rather than containing this tirade in my own head, I direct it at anyone who will listen. Of course, usually my only audience is my children. Fortunately, if I am mindful enough to catch their initial reactions to my tantrum, I can recognize the mess I have created with my struggle against reality and move toward acceptance: This is how it is right now.

Similarly, when we are in a moment of fear or anxiety, sadness, anger, or confusion, often we struggle against that state: "I don't want to feel this way. I can't stand this. Why is this happening again? It's not fair that I get so uncomfortable in these situations." In those moments, acceptance means letting go of the struggle against what is happening in the moment and allowing it to be as it is. Sometimes no action is required beyond acceptance. If Kyle is sitting outside of his doctor's office, waiting to get the results of his stress test, he is likely to feel anxious. The only choice Kyle has in that moment is to struggle against the anxiety or allow it to be. Kyle will feel anxious either way, but if he struggles, he is guaranteed to feel muddy distress as well. On the other hand, sometimes acceptance of an emotional state is needed so that an appropriate action can occur. Jayne sits across the desk from her boss, Frank, who is angrily berating her for requesting a second vacation day this month. She feels some stirrings of anger and fear as her boss's voice gets louder and he starts using obscenities. At first, Jayne struggles against accepting her emotions. "Frank is right—things are really busy right now. A true team player wouldn't let the group down by taking a day off. I have no right to be angry, and what am I afraid of?" Jayne thinks, "Frank is a respected businessman; he is not going to physically hurt me. I'm just being silly." The reality is that no employee deserves to be screamed or sworn at, and angry, out-of-control people can be physically aggressive. For Jayne to remain safe, she needs to acknowledge and accept her emotions so that she can respond to their valid message. Acceptance involves being open to having your experience as it unfolds, without trying to manipulate it, avoid it, escape it, or necessarily change it.

Willingness essentially combines acceptance with engagement in values-consistent behavior. In other words, we are willing when we move forward with an activity that is important to us—like asking someone on a date, saying we are sorry, bringing up a contradictory point, taking on a challenge—even though doing so brings up some painful thoughts or emotions like anxiety or fear. Maggie demonstrates her willingness to engage in a healthy lifestyle by attending a Zumba class even though she has thoughts like "People think I'm too fat and old to be here" and

"I'm uncoordinated and out of breath." She is willing to feel some pain and exertion as she gently pushes her body to take on the physical challenges of the class. She is willing to feel emotions like fear and embarrassment as she tries her best to follow along with the instructor. Similarly, Bob values having a close, honest, and intimate relationship with his wife, Annie, and thus is willing to tell her that her lack of interest in sex makes him feel unattractive. He is willing to feel the discomfort of admitting his vulnerabilities, and he is willing to risk that she might be angry in response.

Sometimes it's easiest to explain what willingness is by clarifying what willingness is not.

Willingness Is Not Wanting

As psychologists who study anxiety, fear, and other emotions, we have developed an appreciation for the value of emotion in human life. An undeniable truth of human existence is that to get the good stuff like love, joy, and surprise you must be willing to experience the painful stuff like sadness, anger, and fear. However, being willing to experience the full range of human emotions is not the same as wanting to do so.

We are not trying to suggest that there is something inherently noble or worthwhile about purposely seeking out difficult thoughts and emotions. Or that one should intentionally approach pain with the goal of becoming a better person. The truth is that if we knew a way to experience all the things we personally value (love, intimacy, friendship, a rewarding career, etc.) without experiencing pain, fear, anxiety, and other uncomfortable emotions, we would choose that option in an instant (and probably write a book about it). There is nothing inherently valuable about feeling pain. Taking a stance of willingness suggests that you will accept and move forward with the thoughts and feelings (rational or irrational) that appear as you make your way through life, taking the actions that will help you obtain the things that you value. You may not like the feelings, you may wish it could be another way, but you can be willing to experience whatever comes up in order to take a valued action.

It's as if you're headed for a beautiful mountain in the distance and the journey is a personally meaningful and valued experience. As you make your trek toward the mountain, you encounter a disgusting, murky swamp that crosses your path and stretches across the landscape for as far as the eye can see. You may not want to walk through that cold, smelly swamp, and it may not seem fair that you need to do so. People approaching the mountain from other directions don't have to deal with this, but the reality is that for you to stay on course you need to cross it. Willingness involves making the choice to slog through because you decide that the journey to the mountain is worth it to you.

Now, we are not saying that you need to belly flop into the swamp and roll around in it on your way to the mountain. Also, if that swamp is slightly off to the side of the path, there is no need to take a detour just to go through it. Your journey to the mountain is not more mean-ingful just because you waded through a swamp to get there. If your path happens to be swamp-free, enjoy it. But if other obstacles present themselves later in the journey—a boulder here, a burr bush there—be willing to encounter these discomforts to stay on course.

If you have actually ever had the pleasure of crossing through a swamp, you might be thinking, Hey, wait a second. Can I bring my wad-ers to make the journey a little more comfortable? Our response would be "Go right ahead and suit up." If you have a warm jacket and some waterproof boots, there is no need to go through the swamp in your shorts and sneakers. Heck, maybe there is some wood lying nearby and you can fashion a plank to walk over. But being willing means that you are open to the possibility that no matter how much protective gear you wear, you could still slip and fall into the putrid waters. And sometimes you might encounter swamps when you don't have any accoutrements. Our suggestion would be that it's fine to try out different ways of mak-ing your journey across the swamp more comfortable as long as you accept the fact that you may still get wet and you are willing to take that chance because of the value of the journey.

Willingness Is an Action, Not a Feeling

As we discussed in Chapter 8, sometimes we mistakenly think we have to feel a certain way or be in a particular state of mind before taking an action. Just as we don't have to feel energetic to exercise, we don't have to feel willing or have willing thoughts to act willing. I (S. M. O.), for example, have a bit of fear related to dental visits. Pretty much every time I have a dental appointment I am visited by thoughts such as "I can't do this," "I don't want to go through this," and "I think I'll cancel my appointment today," and those thoughts continue to hang around while I'm getting ready, driving to the appointment, and often even during the procedure. I may not feel willing to go to the dentist—my thoughts clearly haven't bought the whole concept of willingness—and yet I can behave in a willing manner.

Willingness Is an All-or-Nothing Concept

Just like you cannot be sort of pregnant, you cannot be kind of, or partially, willing. You're either willing or you're not. If Rita is willing to go to the party she feels anxious about *unless* she starts to blush, she is not willing. If Natasha is willing to feel panicky for a few minutes, but no more than five, she is not willing to experience those sensations.

That is not to say that Erin, who struggles with performance anxiety, needs to audition for "American Idol" on TV to be willing to experience anxiety. We can absolutely place limits on the activities we are willing to engage in. For example, Erin might start out by singing out loud in her room when she is alone in the house. Then she might sing in front of a trusted friend and family member, working herself up to a larger and potentially more critical audience. But no matter how small the step, or how limited the risk, a complete and total willingness to experience whatever thoughts, feelings, and sensations emerge is important. So, if Erin commits to singing alone in her room, willingness means she will do it even if she has anxious thoughts and feelings throughout.

Something we've learned through human and animal research, as well as through our own experiences, is that escaping a situation or terminating an activity at the height of anxiety only strengthens the response. Ahn, who struggles with a fear of heights, decides that she will visit her cousin, who happens to live on the top floor of a 30-floor building in the city. Ahn really enjoys her cousin's company, so she decides she is willing to risk experiencing some anxious feelings, but if she feels a full-blown panic attack coming on, she is leaving. What we know about the physiology of anxiety is that it builds over time as the sympathetic part of our nervous system revs up, but that at the nadir of the response the parasympathetic part of our nervous system kicks in and dampens the response. Although people often feel like their anxiety will grow in intensity until they go crazy, have a heart attack, or die, our physiology doesn't work that way. Being willing to stick with an activity can teach us that fear doesn't stick around forever. It is a transient and self-limiting experience. We can also learn that while it may be uncomfortable to feel afraid or anxious, it will not destroy us or prevent us from doing the things we want to do. However, if Ahn always leaves an anxiety-provoking situation at the height of her anxiety, she will never learn that emotions are not dangerous, and she will learn that escaping anxious situations is associated with strong feelings of relief. That learning makes it more and more likely that she will continue to flee anxiety-provoking situations.

Another consequence of being partially willing is that it stops us from participating in and enjoying the things that matter to us. Imagine that you just moved into a new house and you invited all your friends and neighbors on the block over for a housewarming party. You are so excited to be part of a new community that you ask one of the children in the neighborhood to put a flier in the mailbox of every house on the block. All your friends and neighbors show up, and everyone seems to be enjoying themselves, eating tasty appetizers, listening to your favorite music, and engaging in great conversation. You are basking in the glow of having thrown such an excellent party when you hear the unmistakable nasal, high-pitched whine of your annoying neighbor Joe. Your heart skips a beat as you realize your mistake. Although you said everyone on the block was invited, you never intended to include Joe. Joe is a self-absorbed, obnoxious braggart. He takes about himself incessantly—he has the best job, drives the nicest car, has the greenest lawn and the biggest house. If that were not bad enough, Joe is a constant complainer. The food is too spicy, the music too loud, the weather too humid. Oh, no, you think. Why did he show up? What will I do now?

The reality is that you have a few options to choose from:

One is that you can decide you are unwilling to have Joe at your party. What you need to do is march over there and tell him to go home. But you know from past experience that Joe just doesn't listen. Even if he leaves willingly, he will probably try to sneak back in as soon as you disappear into the crowd. The only way to ensure that he stays out is to park yourself by the door and stand guard.

Another option is to decide you are partially willing to have him there. Maybe you can just try for damage control and minimize the negative effect he has on your party. So you could choose to stay with

Joe, to hang out with him on the back porch away from the crowd, to prevent him from mingling with the other guests. If you decide you are fully or partially unwilling to have Joe at the party, your whole experience at the party changes. In the background you can hear your guests. They are still laughing and chatting, enjoying each other's company. They are eating and drinking and dancing to the music, while here you stand guarding Joe. Not much of a party for you.

Finally, you could choose to be willing to have Joe at the party even though you don't enjoy his company or hold a high opinion of him. You don't have to like him, his voice, his opinions, or his lifestyle. You may be embarrassed by his comments about the food and his loud voice. Your opinion of him, your evaluation of him, is absolutely distinct from your willingness to have him as a guest in your home. Allowing Joe to be at the party doesn't mean you have to hang out with him the whole time he's there. It doesn't mean you can't bring your attention to the people at the party whose company you enjoy more. It just means that you will also have Joe there, and Joe will make himself known at times, and if you want to be at the party you're going to have to be willing to have him there too.

How Can We Cultivate an Accepting and Willing Stance?

If we feel defined by our emotions, thoughts, and physical sensations, rather than viewing them as passing experiences, and judge different internal experiences as undesirable and threatening, it's no wonder we're not willing to have these experiences. To shift toward willingness we need to change the relationship we have with our internal experiences. New information—that anxiety is universal, adaptive, and functional; that thoughts and emotions do not necessarily control behavior; and that control efforts backfire—makes new relationships possible. And in our experience, learning is most effective when the information is provided by other sources (books, teaching) as well as personal experience. Therefore, reading this book is (we hope) helpful, but regular mindfulness practice is extremely useful in promoting a curious and compassionate stance toward your experience.

Practicing mindfulness will help you develop what is sometimes referred to as your "observing self." Stepping back and observing your thoughts, emotions, and bodily sensations rather than being entangled with them makes it possible to monitor your own experience without self-criticism or fear. Through self-monitoring you notice when you first begin to feel fear or anxiety (or another difficult emotion) so that you can intervene earlier and earlier in the clear-emotion → judgment → muddy-emotion cycle. Self-monitoring can also increase your awareness of the

> *It is often helpful to practice each exercise we describe in the book at least a few times before moving to the next.*

strategies you engage in—critically judging your emotions, attempting to control them, and avoiding activities that matter to you—that increase your distress. Noticing how unhelpful these responses are will help you stop responding so reflexively. In addition to continuing to practice the formal and informal mindfulness exercises we have described so far, we encourage you to try the slightly more challenging practices introduced in the following pages. Don't be surprised if you find these new exercises challenging; we certainly do.

The Clouds and Sky

Try the following mindfulness exercise to get a sense of yourself as separate from your passing experiences. You can download an audio recording from the book website or read the description below before your practice.

> Close your eyes … first focusing on your breathing, just noticing your breath as you take it in, it travels through your body and then back out of your body … Noticing how your body feels … Noticing any tension in your body … and gently letting it go …
>
> Now picture yourself lying someplace outside where you can see the sky. You can picture any place that feels comfortable and vivid to you—lying on a raft in a pond, on a blanket in a field, on the deck of a house, any place where you have a clear full view of the sky. Just choose the first place that comes to you, rather than spending a lot of time trying to

find the place that seems best. Any place is great. Imagining yourself, lying comfortably, your body sinking into whatever you're lying on, as you gaze at the sky ... Noticing the sky, and the clouds that hang in the sky, moving across it ... Seeing how the clouds are part of the sky, but they are not the whole sky ... The sky exists behind the clouds ... Imagining that your thoughts and feelings are the clouds in the sky, while your mind is the sky itself ... Seeing your thoughts and feelings gently drifting across the sky ... as you notice thoughts and feelings, placing them in the clouds and noticing them, as they pass across the sky ... Noticing yourself as you become distracted, or immersed in the clouds, losing sight of the sky ... noticing how the clouds can be very light and wispy, or dark and menacing ... noticing how even when the clouds cover the sky, the sky exists behind them ... Noticing moments when your thoughts and feelings feel separate from you ... and moments when they feel the same as you ... picturing the sky behind the clouds and the clouds drifting across the sky ... practicing putting your thoughts and feelings on to the clouds ... noticing the different shapes they take ... the different consistency of the clouds they are on ... when you find yourself feeling part of the clouds, slowly bringing your attention back to the sky behind the clouds and practicing putting your thoughts and emotions on the clouds ...

Becoming Disentangled from Our Thoughts

So far we've discussed how harmful it can be to feel defined by our emotions, especially when we consider particular emotions to be unacceptable in some way. Mindfulness practice can show us how our emotions are separate, passing experiences, just like the clouds that waft across the sky. Unfortunately, we also tend to overidentify with, and overrely on, our thoughts. Most of us operate from the perspective that our thoughts and our mind are one and the same. Just like emotions, however, thoughts are merely events that come and go.

We also tend to trust our thoughts, regarding them more or less as truth. Consider, though, where our thoughts come from. They can be acquired through direct experience, like when we learn by exploring on our own that snow feels cold or steel is strong. Thoughts can also be acquired indirectly, through our interactions with others, like when a parent teaches a child that sticking a fork in an electrical outlet can be dangerous. Or a teacher tells us we have potential. Or a parent tells us a situation is unsafe. Or a boss tells us we are incompetent. We all have thoughts about things we learned in school, from our parents, friends, lovers, strangers, TV programs, books, the Internet, and numerous other sources. We can also generate thoughts from situations we imagine, such as "I will fail at this interview" or "I will be alone forever." We are bombarded every day with new "information" derived from direct experience, interactions with others, and our own minds that is stored as thoughts. These thoughts can resurface at any time, and unfortunately our mind doesn't always categorize information by source or veracity.

Complicating the issue of whether our thoughts are true is that statements of truth and opinion are structured in exactly the same way. "This child is female" and "This child is a brat" sound and look pretty similar in sentence structure, although one is clearly a fact and the other a judgment. Also, you are likely to have more of an emotional reaction to one of the statements than the other.

Consider for a moment the sheer number of thoughts that pass through the mind from moment to moment. It can seem as if they move at warp speed. We don't often take the time even to acknowl-

> *It's easy to equate thoughts with truth when statements of fact—"That child is female"—and of opinion—"That child is a brat"—are structured virtually the same.*

edge their presence, never mind to label thoughts as observations and descriptions versus evaluations or judgments. And yet our emotions, bodily sensations, and behaviors all can be affected by the presence of these thoughts.

Defining yourself by your thoughts and always treating their content as truth, or being fused with your thoughts, can really promote unwillingness. Approaching a challenge like allowing yourself to be vulnerable with your partner or taking a risk at work can bring up thoughts such as "I am going to get hurt; I can't stand this" or "I am weak and incompetent." If those thoughts are treated as true indicators of who you are as a person and what might happen to you if you take the challenge, naturally you will be motivated to avoid the situation. And, if the thoughts do crop up, you will try your hardest either to change their content—"I am the perfect candidate for this project"—or push them away.

In contrast, if you approach your thoughts as a collection of things you have heard, learned, and experienced along the way, that may or may not provide you with useful information, their presence is much less threatening. For example, if Jeb has the thought "I am weak" when he considers talking to his partner about his anxiety, and he is fused with his thoughts, he will likely be unwilling to have the conversation. He may also respond to the thought with fear: "Seeing myself as weak is just another indicator of my problem with self-esteem. If I keep thinking this way, I will never be the secure, confident man I want to be." If Jeb feels troubled and insecure about the appearance of this thought, he will try his best to avoid it.

When Luther has the very same thought, he takes a somewhat curious and self-compassionate stance. "Isn't it interesting that these thoughts pop up every time I think about opening up to someone?" he muses. "In our society, men are supposed to seem strong and invincible. Certainly got that message loud and clear from Dad. But that is not the kind of man I want to be. I value being close with my partner even if it means feeling vulnerable sometimes. Plus, being honest and sharing things with another person is a scary thing to do. Pretty much anyone would have thoughts like these in this situation." Luther's ability to step back and observe his thoughts in a self-compassionate, mindful way allows him more flexibility. He can choose to take his desired action even in the presence of such thoughts.

We Can't Control the Uncontrollable with Thoughts

One reason why it is so difficult to detach our sense of self from the content of our thoughts is the deep respect we have for their power. Most of us give our thoughts an awful lot of credit for helping us solve problems and learn new things. Tapping their power is what many people are attempting to do when they worry: come up with solutions to their problems. Research suggests, however, that this strategy typically is not effective. One reason for this is that most of our worries are about unsolvable, uncontrollable problems. For instance, Tiffany worries constantly about the safety of her children and tries to generate ideas for keeping them safe. While it is true that she may be able to generate some concrete ideas with the potential to enhance their safety (require them to wear bike helmets, buy them age-appropriate toys), the unfortunate truth is she cannot completely protect them. Although it is a scary thought, no parent can keep his or her child completely safe; we don't have that level of control. Not accepting that very painful reality motivates Tiffany to go beyond problem solving and to engage in an endless cycle of worry. By constantly imagining potential calamities, she experiences anxiety when she's with her children, which interferes with her ability to enjoy their time together and also leads her children to feel anxious and uneasy. Becky is also overwhelmed with anxiety and unwilling to accept the reality that she doesn't have total control over the safety and security of her children. To cope with her feelings of helplessness, Becky expends considerable effort on avoiding any reminders that childhood risks even exist. Unfortunately, turning a blind eye to the common childhood dangers stops Becky from engaging in the typical safety precautions most parents take.

> *Worry is a way of trying to harness the power of thoughts to solve the unsolvable problems of life.*

We Can't Use Logic to Solve Problems with No Right Answer

Some problems are unsolvable, and no amount of thinking will give us the power to solve them. Other problems involve weighing the pros and cons of different decisions when there is no "right" answer that can be determined through logical analysis. Bert is the health care proxy charged with making medical decisions for his father, Charlie, who is cognitively incapacitated following a recent stroke. Charlie has several chronic medical conditions, including diabetes, high blood pressure, and emphysema. Despite these difficulties, Charlie is functioning fairly well in his current nursing home. He enjoys visits from his family and friends and participates regularly in recreational therapy. Unfortunately, Charlie was recently diagnosed with throat cancer, and although the oncologist recommended a course of chemotherapy, she suggested that the risks of aggressive radiation therapy could outweigh the benefits. Bert pursued a second opinion and received similar advice, although both oncologists were willing to provide the treatment. Bert's siblings are split in their opinions. His brother urges Bert to consider every treatment at their disposal to prolong Charlie's life, and his sister implores Bert to consider Charlie's pain and suffering. Bert is paralyzed with worry about making the right decision. He constantly seeks the opinion of friends and coworkers and spends much of his free time searching the Internet for answers. He also avoids his siblings for fear that they will press him for his decision. Unfortunately, there is no single correct answer to this dilemma. Many of the life issues we struggle with— should I have a baby, should I take this new job, should I leave this relationship, should I move to this new city—have no "right" answers. When we try to mentally solve or think through these problems as we might approach a complicated math problem, we get entangled in a web of worry. Bert's worry and his constant efforts to find the "right" answer are clearly compounding and intensifying the fear, anxiety, and sadness that naturally occur when a family member is ill. Moreover, Bert's worry is keeping him from spending quality time with Charlie and sharing his sadness with his siblings. He imagines that the "right" answer will keep him from his pain, yet the search for this answer is adding to his distress, rather than reducing it.

We Can't Learn Without Experience

Thoughts are also limited in their ability to teach us new ways of responding in the world. When my (S. M. O.) son was very young, he wanted to play soccer, but I missed the sign-up deadline. When I did finally submit his form, the director of the program told me that there was a waiting list and that my son would likely not be placed on a team unless I volunteered to help out the organization. No stranger to volunteerism, and filled with dread at the thought of having to tell Sam he couldn't play, I willingly scribbled my name on the dotted line without a second thought. After all, I could easily hand out jerseys, cut up orange wedges, and organize photo day just as well as the next parent. Imagine my surprise when I received an e-mail with the roster of the team I would be coaching. To say that I am not athletic is a complete understatement. So, I responded to this challenge the same way I respond to most, through scholarly review and research. I went to the library, bought a book about soccer, and began to voraciously read about how to kick the ball (really, you don't use your toes?), dribble (nothing at all like basketball, no hands allowed), and perform a slide tackle (wouldn't it be easier to just call this tripping?). Although I did an OK job of faking my way through the season, it turns out that one cannot learn how to play soccer just by reading. By the end of the season I could describe in detail exactly the right technique for kicking the ball into the net. Despite my outstanding verbal knowledge, my own clumsy attempts were a source of total embarrassment (to me) or hilarity (to my players).

Thinking through problems or thinking about how to do something can only take us so far. Some things (like soccer) are best learned and known through experience. Think about how babies learn to walk. Parents don't sit down and explain the basic techniques to their children, and there is no instruction video. Children can learn to walk only through direct experience. They pay attention to what works and what doesn't, make minor adjustments, and try again and again.

Thinking Often Interferes with Experiencing

Not only is it the case that experience can teach us things that words or thoughts cannot; it is also true that thoughts can interfere with our ability to learn through experience. Although an athlete develops skill through both verbal coaching (e.g., keep your feet shoulder width apart, maintain a tight two-knuckle overlap grip, pivot on the backswing) and experience, to perform at the top of their game athletes try to achieve a state referred to as *flow*. Flow (similar to mindfulness) is the mental state of being totally immersed in the present moment. It requires that the athlete move from a state of self-consciousness to one in which she is absorbed in the activity. Overthinking prevents flow or often diminishes performance.

Being lost in thought can also prevent us from fully engaging with and learning from the events going on around us. Whether the thoughts are about the task you are trying to learn ("I am so stupid—why can't I figure out how to use this computer program?") or something else ("I am so worried about how we will make our next mortgage payment"), their hold on our attention prevents us from fully benefiting from experience.

Humans benefit tremendously from the ability to think. Yet to reap the most benefit from this wonderful and unique ability, we need to recognize thoughts for what they are.

EXERCISE **Labeling thoughts as thoughts**

One small change you can make that will begin to help you change your relationship with your thoughts is to label thoughts for what they are—both in your mind and in the way you speak, if you are willing. For example, if your child is misbehaving and you have the thought "I am a horrible parent," we would like you to try to catch yourself and rephrase that as "I am having the thought or evaluation that I am a horrible parent." Perhaps you are a horrible parent. Or maybe in that moment you have that thought because you are tired, overwhelmed, and your daughter doesn't appreciate the fact that you set some limits. Or it could be that usually you are a pretty good parent and you had a less than stellar parenting moment. If you are asked to work overtime and you don't want to, notice your instinct to think "I can't say no" and consider "I am having the thought that I cannot say no." Maybe you would be fired on the spot if you said no. Or perhaps your boss wouldn't be happy about it, but there wouldn't be any consequences. Or maybe your boss would be fine with your turning down overtime. Placing "I am having the thought" before a thought is simply a reminder to slow down and consider the source and accuracy of its content.

Although our focus here is thoughts, we encourage you to use this convention with all your internal experiences, as part of your mindfulness practice. When you notice "I am anxious," you might consider "I am having some anxious feelings." If you start thinking about how poorly an interaction with your partner might go, try describing your experience as "my mind is imagining he will get angry and not listen to me." When you feel short of breath, notice "my breathing pattern has shifted to being rapid and shallow."

Another mental and verbal shorthand we frequently engage in without much attention or awareness is to provide motivation for our behavior. Specifically, we often use thoughts, feelings, and emotional responses as reasons for a particular behavior. The problem is that sometimes when we give reasons for our behavior, although the reasons may sound like facts, they may actually reflect judgments and/or choices that are often hidden or difficult to see. For instance, we might easily say that we did not accept a dinner invitation because we were too anxious, when in fact one could choose to dine out even while extremely anxious. Anxiety and fear may prompt us to avoid, but they do not force us to. We are still physically capable of following through with an action that is inconsistent with a feeling. The problem is that our reasoning happens so quickly that we just accept it at face value and do not even notice the assumption inherent in our reasoning (i.e., that we cannot do something if we will be anxious doing it).

EXERCISE **Rethinking but**

Many times we say we would like to do something *but* there is some reason that we cannot. For instance, I want to go shopping, *but* I am anxious. Try to catch yourself every time you think or say *but* and see if the statement is accurate if *but* is replaced with *and*. *But* sometimes suggests that the second part of the statement (I am anxious) is more important than the first (I want to go shopping). *And* suggests that both parts of the statement are accurate.

Mindfulness of Thoughts

Practicing mindfulness of thoughts can be both challenging and rewarding. There are several variations that you can try. Your task is to visualize your thoughts one after another as you become aware of them.

Some people find it useful to place each thought on a leaf and watch it flow by on a stream. Others prefer to imagine thoughts appearing and passing by on a movie screen. You may want to try a few options to find an image that works for you. Any thought you have, like "This seems really silly," "I wonder what's for lunch," or "I wish I wasn't so anxious," can be observed, one after another. The purpose of the exercise is to notice each time you shift from looking *at* your thoughts to looking *from* your thoughts. You will know that has happened when you realize you stopped paying attention to the exercise and got caught in your thoughts.

It's very unlikely that you'll be able observe your thoughts for very long without interruption. When you do notice that you have stopped participating or lost the point of the exercise, back up a few seconds and see whether you can catch what you were doing right before you stopped observing your thoughts. Then go ahead and slip back into observing mode. If you have trouble getting started and think "I am not having any thoughts at all," or "It's not working," or "I'm not doing it right," those would be good thoughts to observe.

Accepting Means Turning Toward, Not Another Way to Turn Away From

As you begin to practice accepting your internal responses, you may notice that sometimes distressing thoughts or feelings become less intense or dissipate completely when you turn toward them. Naturally, people often enjoy this potential effect of acceptance and begin to practice acceptance as a way of getting rid of anxious thoughts or feelings. It's easy to find ourselves vigorously trying to put anxious thoughts on a leaf and wishing the stream would quickly carry them away so they wouldn't bother us again. And yet, this brings us back to the cycle of trying to get rid of our feelings described in Chapter 8 and will undoubtedly backfire. Sometimes acceptance will lead thoughts or feelings to pass quickly; sometimes it will lead us to feel pain more deeply before we learn what it's teaching us so that we can move forward in our lives. While it's perfectly human to hope for the former outcome rather than the latter, it's important to be open to either and to turn toward our experience rather than away from it.

Ivan had been experiencing anxiety and worry for years when he decided to seek therapy to try addressing it. He enjoyed the mindfulness exercises he did with his therapist and practiced at home because he often found that his mind quieted and he didn't have so many racing thoughts of potential catastrophes. He liked the idea of trying not to get entangled in his thoughts and tried to apply it in his life. When he began to worry that his teenage son, Nick, seemed distant from him, he told himself not to get "caught up in" his worries and tried to focus on other things. Each time he interacted with Nick, he would notice that Nick avoided his gaze and didn't answer his questions directly. Ivan's chest would tighten as he wondered what was wrong with his son. Noticing this response, Ivan would again urge himself not to get "caught up in" these concerns and he would turn his attention away from Nick and toward something else like the food he was eating or a TV show they were watching.

When Ivan talked about this situation with his therapist, he reiterated his intention to accept his response and not get caught up in it by moving on to other things. Although he reported that it was helping, Ivan seemed on edge and uncomfortable as he discussed his concerns about Nick. His therapist asked him what it would be like to turn toward these feelings, rather than focusing on not getting caught up in them. After some time, Ivan was able to experience the sadness underlying his worries about Nick and to notice his desire to reach out to Nick in some way. Although this realization was painful, it was ultimately satisfying because it helped him to truly accept his response and to learn what his emotions were telling him.

EXERCISE **First and second reactions**

So far, we have asked you to use mindfulness in all of the monitoring exercises to bring a new awareness to your reactions. We have asked you to observe anxiety-provoking situations, to notice the full range of thoughts and feelings that emerge, and to become aware of your urges to control internal pain. We hope that monitoring has made you become more aware of your experiences. From this point forward, we are going to suggest that you bring the full range of mindfulness skills to your monitoring. As always, when you notice anxiety, worry, or any other painful emotions or thoughts arise, make an entry in your notebook. Note the date and situation, the first set of reactions that arise (e.g., clear emotions), and the reaction you have to your reactions. In other words, were you judgmental and critical? Did you try to control your reaction? Or did you bring acceptance and willingness? Were you self-compassionate? Finally, jot down your behavioral reactions. Did you stay in the situations? Snap at someone? Shut down? Tell the person how you really felt? Did you breathe? Monitoring can be a concrete way to help you develop a new habit, the mindfulness habit, to responding to reactions. We suggest that you continue monitoring in this way until you feel a new habit has been established.

10

clarifying what matters to you and setting a course for change

Darcy listened to the sound of the New Year's Eve party down the hall in her apartment building and tried to ignore the texts she kept receiving from her friends, asking when she'd be arriving at their friend's party. She imagined them all there and tried to picture herself going. Her breathing became shallow as she imagined the people she wouldn't know and how crowded the rooms would be. Her heart began racing and she felt dizzy. She took a deep breath and turned off her phone and turned up the TV while she tried to decide which frozen dinner to heat up. She couldn't go to the party; she knew she would have a panic attack if she went. She tried to focus on the TV program, but her mind kept returning to the party she was missing. She tried to think of resolutions for the coming year. All that came to mind is that she wanted not to be so anxious.

Many people who come to see us for help with anxiety, like Darcy, can't think of what they want in their lives, other than that they don't want to be anxious. Other people can think of things they wish they were doing—being open in their relationships or being open to new relationships, living a healthy life, doing creative work, or making contributions to their community—but believe the anxiety they experience makes these things impossible. Some people can think of ways they wish other people lived their lives differently and feel frustrated by their inability to change those people. Others are doing things that matter to them, yet they feel like they *should* be living differently. Still others are living in ways that are meaningful and important but feel like spectators in their lives and do not experience the benefits of these full lives. Regardless of which of these descriptions matches you best (or perhaps your experience is completely different but you know anxiety gets in the way of living the life you want to be living), an important step in cultivating a different way of being in your life is clarifying what really matters to you.

As discussed in the last few chapters, and as you know from your own experience, getting rid of anxiety is not as easy as it sounds. And efforts to get rid of it can make it worse. We have introduced the alternative of being willing to experience whatever arises in the moment, including anxiety and distress, and you've been developing mindfulness and other skills to help you be willing. However, remember that an essential part of willingness is that we are willing because having these experiences allows us to move toward something that matters to us. In the swamp metaphor introduced in the last chapter, we don't go through the swamp when it isn't between us and the mountain—yet we are willing to go through the muck when it lies along our path to something we value.

Unfortunately, we can easily become distracted from what we value or what matters to us as we try to avoid feeling distress. Often we develop a habit of ignoring the things that matter to us as we try to feel more comfortable and certain in our lives. Without a clear sense of what is important, we cannot make choices based on moving toward what matters, and so we habitually choose instead to move away from anxiety or distress. Yet, as we have already explored together, this habitual moving away from pain does not lead us to avoid pain at all (in fact, quite the opposite).

The exercises and practices you have done up until now have helped you turn toward your emotions instead of avoiding them and cultivate a different relationship with your thoughts and emotions so that you can choose your actions rather than reacting. In this chapter, we introduce exercises to help you explore and identify what matters to you (or what you *value*) so your values can inform your choices and allow you to live the life you want to be living. What matters to you may already have become clearer as you have been practicing mindfulness and bringing more awareness to your life in general. Nonetheless, you may find that the exercises in this chapter illuminate or clarify values you haven't thought about lately and that may help you guide your life.

What Do We Mean by *Values*?

We use the term *values* in a very specific way, which may not be the first meaning that comes to mind when you hear the word. We do not mean prescriptions that come from some external source about what we *should* do, or morals. We mean identifying what we ourselves think is important or meaningful—what we personally value. There are no right or wrong values, and each person's values will differ from another's. One person may value being emotionally open in relationships, while another may value being truthful, and a third may value being kind. As long as we each recognize what matters to us, we can make choices consistent with these values as we navigate our lives.

How Values Differ from Goals

If values are what we want out of life, you may wonder whether what we're talking about is really just goals. But there's an important difference. Take a moment to think about your current or past goals. Have you ever wanted to lose weight, to meet someone special, or get promoted at work? Goals like these can be helpful and motivating and can lead to behavior change. But what if we don't achieve them? Most of us have set goals, failed to meet them, and then felt discouraged and given up efforts to change those aspects of our lives. Even setting a goal can make you feel discontent with the present. Goals always point to the future, so they indicate that something about the present is unsatisfactory. Focusing on a goal can make us feel bad about how things are in the moment and can lead us to imagine that all will be well when we reach this future goal (which usually turns out not to be the case). Goals can make us less accepting of our current circumstances—our current weight, single status, less ideal job—in a way that reduces our compassion for ourselves. Also, it is not always very satisfying or enriching to work toward goals, particularly if we believe we might not be able to attain them.

By reducing our compassion for ourselves and focusing our attention on a destination that we believe we have to reach—but might not—goals can actually contribute to anxiety.

None of this is to say that we shouldn't set goals; they can be important planning tools, if nothing else. But without values guiding what we do in the moment, they might be empty, misleading, or disappointing. Values refer to a process, a direction, rather than an outcome. We can engage our values in the present, letting them inform every moment. Goals, in contrast, are always future focused, an endpoint. If you value taking care of your physical well-being, you can eat a healthy meal and exercise today even though weight loss won't occur right away. You can intimately connect with people in your life right now, even if you're not dating anyone. You can complete your work efficiently and effectively and even propose a new process for your unit to consider, even though you may wish for a more challenging and responsible position. Values allow us to behave in ways that are important to us in the moment and to reap the immediate rewards of an enhanced life. Whether they are met or not, goals expire.

One way to illustrate this distinction is through this metaphor. Suppose you really enjoy downhill skiing and you plan a trip for weeks. The day of your ski trip arrives; you purchase your lift ticket, wait in line, and finally arrive at the top of the hill. As you are about to push off, someone steps up and asks you about your goal: "Where are you trying to get to?" the man asks. When you reply "the bottom of the hill," he insists he can help you attain that goal and promptly hustles you into a helicopter, flies you to the bottom of the hill, and then disappears. Consider how you might feel. Although the goal of skiing is to get to the bottom of the hill, the fun is in the process. Having the goal of getting to the bottom is important, because it allows you to engage in the process. But the value in skiing is the swooshing down the powdered hill.

It is similar to falling in love. Imagine that your goal is to commit to a life partner. You attend a party, and all of a sudden you catch the eye of an attractive and engaging man or woman across the room. Magically, your life fast-forwards through the process and ends at the moment you achieve your goal. Next thing you know, you are walking away with this man or woman who is now your life partner. You got to skip the awkward moments, the first fight, meeting your in-laws. However, you also skipped the anticipation of the first kiss, the warm glow that accompanies feelings of true connection, the moments when you first shared vulnerable feelings and memories, and the experience of celebrating your love in whatever way you both find meaningful during a wedding or commitment ceremony.

Goals can point us in valued directions, but values are the underlying force that guides us in setting goals and working toward them. Values bring dignity to our actions in the present moment. If we value openness in our relationships, we can choose to open up to someone in our lives today, in some way, even if we aren't yet in the intimate relationship we would like to be in. For one person "being open" might mean connecting with a good friend over dinner, for another it might

> *Acting on values can bring fulfillment and meaning into our lives in every moment.*

be chatting with someone on Facebook, and still another person can value openness by conversing with a coworker for a few minutes when she usually hides in her cubicle. Acting on values can immediately bring moments of fulfillment and meaning into our lives, particularly if we are mindful of our actions.

On the other hand, we can sometimes meet our goals and not behave in ways that are consistent with our values. For example, one might achieve the goal of being in a committed relationship but not have open and honest communication. Or one can lose weight through extremely unhealthy actions. Achieving goals in the absence of value-guided actions often leaves us feeling discontent or dissatisfied. So goals can be helpful, but clarifying our values and acting in ways that are consistent with those values can deepen and enhance our lives.

Now that you have a better sense of what we mean by values, we would like you to take some time to clarify your personal values. We recommend taking a break from reading to complete this exercise over the next few days and then reading the rest of the chapter after you have finished the exercise.

EXERCISE **Exploring your personal values**

At the end of Chapter 2 we asked you to write about how anxiety and avoidance were affecting and limiting three areas of your life: relationships, work/school/household management, and self-nurturance/

community involvement. We would like you to read over your responses to that exercise before you begin this exercise, in which we will continue to look at these three areas of living to identify what matters to you in each of them.

Please set aside 20 minutes on three different days during which you can privately and comfortably do this writing assignment. Once again, in your writing we want you to really let go and explore your very deepest emotions and thoughts about the topics listed below. You may want to take several minutes to practice mindfulness before you start, so that you can approach this task with open-hearted awareness.

As you write, try to allow yourself to experience your thoughts and feelings as completely as you can. As we've discussed, pushing these disturbing thoughts away can actually make them worse, so try to really let yourself go. Bring your mindfulness practice to the exercise so that you can accept and allow any reactions you have and continue to clarify what matters to you most. If you cannot think of what to write next, repeat the same thing over and over until something new comes to you. Be sure to write for the entire 20 minutes. Don't be concerned with spelling, punctuation, or grammar; just write whatever comes to mind.

You may notice that you often have thoughts about why you cannot be the way you would like to be in a particular area. This is natural and is why we asked you about the obstacles to your values in these areas in the earlier writing exercise. We continue to explore these obstacles in the following chapter. So, for this particular exercise, see if you can notice these thoughts as they arise and gently turn your attention back to how you would like to be if you were not experiencing the obstacle so that you can really explore what matters to you.

DAY 1: RELATIONSHIPS

Choose two or three relationships that are important to you. You can either pick actual relationships (e.g., my relationship with my brother) or relationships you would like to have (e.g., I would like to be part of a couple, I would like to make more friends). Briefly write about how you would like to be in those relationships. Think about how you would like to *communicate with others* (e.g., how open vs. private you would like to be, how direct vs. passive you would like to be in asking for what you need and in giving feedback to others). Think about *what sort of support you would like* from other people and *what sort of support you can give* without sacrificing your self-care. Write about anything else that matters to you in your relationships with others.

DAY 2: WORK/ EDUCATION/HOUSEHOLD MANAGEMENT

Briefly write about the sort of work, training, education, or household management you would like to be engaged in and *why that appeals to you.* Next write about *the kind of worker and/or student and/or household manager* you would like to be with respect to your work habits and your *relationships* with your boss/coworkers, or classmates. What is important to you about the *product of your work/studies?* How would you like to *communicate to others* about your work? How would you like to *respond to feedback?* Are there additional *challenges* you would like to take on? Write about anything else that matters to you in this area.

DAY 3: SELF-NURTURANCE AND COMMUNITY INVOLVEMENT

Write about how you would like to *spend your free time,* whether you actually have any free time in your life right now. What would you like to do to have *fun?* What types of activities do you feel *feed or nurture you?* How could you *take better care of yourself* (e.g., nutrition, exercise, spirituality)? Are there ways you would like to be more *involved with your community?* Write about anything else that matters to you in this area of living.

You may be wondering why we consistently refer to these three domains throughout the book. We have found in our own lives and working with clients that it is helpful to attend to the full range of our lives when we try to make changes. Otherwise, we run the risk of having changes in one area of life hinder our valued actions in another area. So, we suggest that you keep all three domains in your awareness as you continue through the exercises in the rest of the book. You may feel like you are already living a full life in one domain, such as work, yet need to focus on what matters to you in another, such as community involvement. Nonetheless, by focusing on both you may find that there are some actions you take at work that are not as valued and may take you away from your community involvement. Keeping all three in mind can help with making these kinds of adjustments.

Clarifying What Matters to You

Now that you have spent some time thinking about what matters to you, you have taken an important step toward clarifying the choices you want to make in your life and the directions you want to move in. For all of us, this clarification is an ongoing process, and many questions may arise as we carefully examine what seems to be important to us. The following sections present some things to consider as you refine your values to determine the direction you want to go in. In Chapter 11, we explore how you can engage in actions consistent with these values, using the mindfulness skills you have been developing throughout this book.

Letting Actions Lead and Feelings Follow

For many of us, our immediate answers to the question of how we want to be living our lives refer to how we want to *feel* in our lives, rather than what we want to *do*. Like Darcy, who could only desire a life in which she did not experience anxiety, we may find ourselves wishing we felt happy more often, or felt self-confident with new people, or felt calm in the face of stress. These are very natural responses. We often believe we need to feel a certain way (e.g., courageous or confident) to do things (e.g., go on a first date or apply for a new job). However, this is not actually the case. And we've already examined how emotions are natural, human responses and that trying to feel certain ways and not feel other ways doesn't work and can actually leave us feeling worse. It can be very painful to wish that things were other than they

> *We can do things that matter to us even if we feel anxious while doing them.*

are. So, it may be worthwhile to try a different path—letting our actions lead and our feelings follow, rather than the other way around.

People are often surprised by the idea of doing something regardless of how they feel. As we discussed in Chapter 8, we all tend to believe that feelings have to come before actions. But, in fact, we can do anything at any time, regardless of how we feel. This is actually a central idea in one form of effective therapy for depression. People experiencing depression often feel unmotivated to do things they used to enjoy—and don't get much enjoyment when they do them. So they stop doing these things, which further contributes to their depression. But extensive research shows that engaging in actions they used to enjoy improves their satisfaction with their lives and even their moods. Our feelings can follow our actions instead of preceding them. This gives us a lot more freedom and flexibility in our lives because we don't have to wait until we feel a particular way to do something important to us.

The concept of self-confidence provides another example of how our usual way of thinking can be misleading. People often think of self-confidence as a state in which a person has no self-doubt, fear, or negative self-evaluations. It is probably more accurate (and useful) to think of self-confidence as trusting or having faith in oneself, even in the face of fear. So we can feel uncertain, doubtful, and frightened and still act in ways that demonstrate self-confidence or faith (such as asserting ourselves at work or introducing ourselves to someone new). This is similar to courage, which means acting while one is scared, not acting without fear. Doing something without the experience of fear really isn't very challenging at all—courage and strength are evident when we experience fear and still pursue something that matters to us.

Look back over your writing from the past several days and see if you wrote about how you want to feel rather than what you want to do. If you did, take some time to think about how you would live your life differently if you did feel calm, or self-confident, or happy. What kind of work would you do if you felt confident? What would you be like in relationships if you felt courageous? If you imagine yourself in the emotional state you are hoping for, what kinds of actions would you be taking that you aren't taking now? Make a list in your notebook of the things you would be doing if you felt the way you want to feel. Then look back over the list and see which of these are things that deeply matter to you. Put an asterisk next to each action that represents a valued direction.

EXERCISE **Who is driving your bus?**

People often have trouble imagining what it would be like to choose actions regardless of how they are feeling or thinking. The mindfulness

practices you have been doing will help you experience your thoughts and feelings as rising and falling, rather than as such defining experiences that you have to follow where they lead you. As you explore the directions you want to be moving in, you will likely have thoughts and feelings that suggest these directions are not possible for you. Try the clouds and sky mindfulness exercise or the mindfulness of thoughts exercises from Chapter 9 to help you get a little bit of distance between yourself and your internal experiences so that you can more easily take actions that matter to you regardless of how you are feeling in the moment.

Another exercise that can help is to imagine you're driving a bus and the thoughts, feelings, and sensations you have are passengers. You're driving along a route that reflects your valued direction. But these passengers in the back represent your worries, sensations of anxiety, feelings of dread, thoughts that you are not capable of doing certain things, or any other internal experience that is getting between you and where you want to go. As you drive along, following your route, these passengers may start threatening you and telling you where to go: "You have got to turn left," "You have to turn right here," and so on. They speak with authority, and they are frightening and menacing, as we know our internal experiences can be. The threat is if you don't do what they say, they are going to come up to the front of the bus.

As we have already explored together, it is natural and human not to want to see these painful experiences up close. So we often make a deal with these passengers that we will go wherever they say, as long as they scrunch down in the back so we cannot see them clearly and don't have to fully experience the thoughts and feelings they represent. But, of course, then we aren't driving in the direction we value.

Another option people sometimes take is to decide to go to the back and deal with those passengers. They pull over their metaphorical bus and focus solely on trying to deal with the difficult thoughts and feelings so that they can then go on to live a fulfilling life. But to do this they have to park the bus, so they are no longer driving their route and following their valued direction. And the passengers aren't dealt with easily. As you saw in Chapter 8, we cannot actually make them go away by trying.

The solution, then, is to drive the bus and let the passengers shout all they want. We can use our mindfulness skills to notice the thoughts and feelings as they are—"There's a thought that I can't possibly succeed at this," "There are feelings of anxiety and dread"—and just keep driving in the direction we choose. Sometimes the noise may be almost deafening as the passengers try to get us to go a different way. We can take a breath, notice our experience, remember what matters to us, and continue on our path. Sometimes we may find that we failed to notice the passengers had taken over and that we have turned in the direction they chose for us. That's natural. When we notice this, we can smile at how forceful those passengers can be, feel compassion for the challenge that faces us as we continue on our route with particularly unruly passengers on this day, and find our way back to our chosen route. The more we practice choosing our actions, the easier it is for us to notice when we have strayed from our route and to return to following our valued direction. Over time we may find that simply asking ourselves "Who is driving my bus?" is a way to return to valued action when we have moved off course.

Personal Preference or Avoidance?

J.D. listened while the guys he worked with made plans to head to a bar after work to watch the game. When someone asked if he wanted to join them, he politely declined. He thought about how different he was from them—they all seemed to really enjoy being around people and made a lot of plans to get together outside of work. He had never been a "people person." He enjoyed his solitary routines, the quiet of his apartment where he lived alone, the predictability of relying on himself rather than on other people. As he heard his coworkers laughing together, he felt a pang of envy and a slight feeling of sadness. He quickly brushed them off and imagined how nice it would be to just relax at home alone, eat what he wanted to eat, and not have to worry about anyone else.

When we develop strong habits of avoiding things that make us anxious, it can be very difficult to tell whether we do certain things because we prefer them or because we're avoiding another option. People with an apparently strong preference to be around people are sometimes avoiding being alone, while those who describe themselves as solitary may be minimizing the anxiety they experience when they are with people. Someone who constantly changes jobs and locations may truly enjoy variety and new challenges, or she may instead be avoiding fears of making a commitment to one place or one job. And, of course, often our apparent preferences are a combination of a true preference and avoidance of fears or distress. J.D. may in fact really enjoy the silence and solitude of his apartment, and it may be important for him to spend time alone. Yet he may also yearn to have more social contact, and he may not be noticing these desires because he is so convinced that he is not a "people person."

> *Being rigid about our choices usually indicates avoidance, while flexibility is a sign of preference.*

One way to tell whether our preferences are guided by avoidance is to think about how rigid and stuck to them we are. If we never get on the highway, even when sticking to the back roads causes significant inconvenience, we are probably avoiding driving on the highway. If, on the other hand, we will take the highway when necessary, but choose to take back roads when time is not an issue, we may truly prefer driving on the back roads. Flexible behavior that varies based on the specific context is often

> *Are we choosing something because we really want it—or because we feel anxiety about the alternative?*

an indication of choice and preference, while rigid behavior that is the same across multiple situations and contexts frequently reflects efforts to avoid pain or distress. Bringing mindful awareness to our actions can help us notice whether the things we are doing truly reflect our preferences.

EXERCISE **Avoidance or personal preference?**

Take a few moments to look through your values writing and see if you wrote about values that may actually be, at least in part, driven by avoidance. It may help to bring mindfulness to this task—first focusing on your breathing, and then allowing any thoughts or emotions to arise as you look through your values writing. You may want to make a list of things you prefer in each domain and then rate how much these reflect a preference and how much they reflect avoidance on a 100-point scale. So if you like to work alone, really think about working alone and how satisfying that is for you. Then think about working with other people and whether that is actually unappealing or raises anxiety and that is what makes it unappealing to you. Imagine working with other people and notice the reactions that arise. If avoidance of discomfort is present, rate the level of that avoidance on a scale of 0 to 100, so that you can begin to get a sense of how much your choices are efforts to move away from one option, rather than moving toward something you truly prefer. Make a list of those actions that reflect true personal preferences. Make a separate list of actions that might seem like preferences but that you now think may be driven more by avoidance. You can pay attention to times when you feel drawn to engage in these actions and choose instead to follow true preferences in these contexts.

Separating Our Values from the Values of Other People

The people who are central in our lives often influence what seems important to us. This is natural—we learn what kind of person, student, or worker we want to be, how to be in relationships, and how to spend our free time from the example (and sometimes instruction) of those who raise us and those we admire. Over the course of our lives, these values may have changed as we realize that some things our parents or other caregivers valued are not as important to us, while other things that they discounted actually matter quite a bit to us. We may meet new people who care about different things and find that some of them matter to us as well—we just hadn't considered them before.

Throughout this natural process of refining your personal values and allowing them to change as you grow, you may find yourself confused because you just instinctively take on certain values (perhaps those of a partner you love a great deal) or continue to hold long-standing values (like those learned from parents or caregivers) when they don't match your own personal sense of what is important. This is a challenging position to be in, because it may lead you to choose actions that leave you feeling dissatisfied and unfulfilled because the actions weren't based on your own true values.

A good indicator that your values are reflections of someone else's rather than your own personal sense of meaning and importance is when they sound like rules or *should* statements, rather than expressions of your own sense of what matters.

EXERCISE **Identifying your *own* personal values**

Take some time to look back through your values writing from the last several days and see whether any of the values you wrote about come from someone else in your life and do not truly reflect your own values. If you can hear someone else saying something you wrote about, it may not be your own value. Use your mindfulness skills to really notice your true response to the potential value to see if it matters to you. You may want to take some time to focus on your breathing and then notice the thoughts, emotions, images, and memories that arise as you read over each value. Notice whatever arises for you, allowing it to come without judging it. See whether some of the values you listed are really tied to other people and don't reflect your own preferences. List any values that seem to come from someone else separately so that you can be aware that you may feel pulled to act according to these values at times, yet they are unlikely to be satisfying to you. Then list those values that you truly feel inside are important, with asterisks, to continue to develop your understanding of what really matters to you. If you have trouble telling whether a value comes from you or someone else, take some time to notice what arises when you think of the value, continuing to breathe, allowing any responses to arise, without judgment. If it still isn't clear, list these values under a question mark and continue to bring attention to them throughout your daily life. Over time it will become clearer whether these are truly your personal values or something you inherited from someone else.

Wanda worked as an editor and freelance writer at a literary magazine. She was single and had a number of very good friends. Wanda's parents had always been very enthusiastic about her writing and were certain she was destined for a brilliant writing career. They also longed for grandchildren and often talked about what a wonderful mother Wanda would be. Wanda had shared these

values with them while growing up, yet recently she found her-
self struggling to determine whether they reflected her own values.
Although Wanda forced herself to devote a block of time to writing
each weekend, she began to feel as if she were just going through
the motions. Several weekends in a row, Wanda canceled her plans
with her good friends at the last minute to accept a date with a
man she had recently met through her parents. Although he was
kind and funny, Wanda didn't feel a deep connection or attraction
to him, and she missed spending time with her friends. Wanda
felt confused and discouraged because although she was actively
taking steps to pursue these life directions, she felt dissatisfied and
unfulfilled much of the time. When she went through the process
of clarifying her values described above, and really started pay-
ing attention to her experiences and responses, she realized that
she had a real talent for helping authors find ways to effectively
communicate what they were trying to say and felt genuine sat-
isfaction in the process of shaping a rough story into a beautifully
written gem. She no longer wanted to write herself, because she
found editing more satisfying. She also realized that deep emotional
connections were more important to her than being in a committed
relationship and that she missed the time she used to spend with
her friends. She chose to end her current relationship to be in more
fulfilling relationships, even though that meant she was not cur-
rently moving toward a committed relationship and children. She
remained unsure whether she truly wanted children and planned
to keep paying attention to whether this was a valued direction or
not.

Wanda was living a life guided by her own values, but also was sticking to old values that came in part from her parents. Bringing awareness
to the satisfaction we experience in response to different actions can
help us identify what truly matters to us, rather than what we think
should matter to us. Of course, acting in ways that are consistent with
our values does not always feel comfortable or easy. If you value being
open in relationships, you will undoubtedly experience the full range of
emotions—sadness, anger, fear, joy—in the process. Valuing a healthy
lifestyle can mean learning to tolerate the urge to indulge in a pint of
chocolate ice cream and trudging to the gym on a cold, rainy night

when you might wish to be curled up on a cozy chair at home. It is not the moment-to-moment experience of emotion that indicates the presence or absence of values. Instead, it is a larger sense that we are living with purpose and intent. We are willing to feel and think and experience passing discomfort to participate fully in our lives. Being mindful can really help us notice these distinctions.

Wanting Other People to Act Differently

One of the most painful challenges we face in trying to live a value-guided life is our inability to change how other people act. When you were exploring what's important to you, did you find yourself thinking about how someone else could be different and how that would make your life more meaningful? It's completely reasonable to want a partner to respond with compassion rather than criticism or a boss to notice successes in addition to failures or a neighborhood group to work together more effectively. Many of us find ourselves in situations that seem unfair. A mother-in-law may make demands that are unreasonable and seem impossible to satisfy; a coworker may regularly call attention to her own successes and your failures; a church member may be an ineffective leader but refuse to share the leadership role or take advice. Your emotional responses provide important information about an upsetting context, but they don't necessarily guide you to the actions that will help you. And as you begin to draw attention to your own experiences in each of these contexts, you're likely to find that desperately wanting these people to be different from the way they are is adding to your suffering, rather than addressing it.

Sometimes finding the actions that *will* help you involves taking a specific context into account and deciding the person you want to be in that context. If your partner isn't responding to you as you prefer, you can think about how you want to communicate this desire to your partner or how you might be able to model this behavior yourself. Kara, for example, wishes Michael showed her more affection, so she might tell him how much she likes it when he kisses her on the cheek or holds her hand when they're walking together. (If this is a long-standing issue for the

> *Trying to control the uncontrollable—other people—fans the flames of anxiety and increases our distress.*

couple, mindfulness might help Kara respond with equanimity to the thoughts and emotions that arise before and during the conversation and keep her focused on the present moment.)

Some people find, when they bring beginner's mind to the situation, that perfectly understandable reactions they have contribute to the dynamic and they may want to try to address them. Kara was surprised and a bit embarrassed when Michael pointed out the reaction she often had when he did show affection: "Why are you acting so sweet to me? You must want something, or you must have really screwed up!"

The point is that ultimately we don't have control over anyone else's behavior, including someone as close to us as a partner. If the other person's behavior doesn't change once we've taken actions consistent with our own values, such as being the person we want to be in the relationship or clearly communicating our wishes, we have a choice to make. We may choose to accept the person as-is and give up our struggle to try to make him or her different. Or we may choose to end the relationship.

Our desire to control the behavior of others often muddies our emotions and pulls us toward responses and actions that are inconsistent with our values. And acting in ways that are inconsistent with our values contributes to our personal distress. Recognizing our growing distress and attributing it to the relationship can trigger stronger and more desperate attempts to control the other person. If we are not mindful of these complicated reactions, aware of our own personal values, and accepting of the limits to control, it is very easy to get caught in these distressing interpersonal cycles.

For example, if Rex senses that Carla is losing interest in him, he may begin to search for things he can say or do to hold on to the relationship. He might give up some of his own interests, like volunteering at his church and playing basketball with his friends after work, to help her with errands and chores around her apartment. If Carla doesn't return Rex's calls for 2 weeks in a row, he might leave a string of desperate messages begging her to stay with him. Or he might post cheery false status messages on his Facebook page to give the illusion that he doesn't care about her at all. All of these actions are aimed at changing the attraction Carla feels for Rex, something he has limited control over. None of them are consistent with his own values. So each behavior brings double distress—it makes Rex feel out of control and ineffective.

It can be difficult to recognize these patterns and to let go of the struggle of trying to control the important people in our lives. One particularly challenging situation arises when we feel that we would be giving in or showing weakness if we were to act kind or reasonable toward someone who treats us poorly. If we sense we are being treated unjustly, we might respond by treating the other person badly to even the playing field. While it seems like such actions would make us feel strong and satisfied, they often backfire and leave us feeling angry, resentful, and confused.

Rod and George have been working in the same office for 10 years, and they are polar opposites in personality. They don't see eye to eye on any issue, and they are frequently embroiled in battle. In the early days, the manager had tried to intervene, but the men were so set in their ways, unwilling to listen or make any concessions, that he just gave up and tried his best to keep them apart. After one particularly painful staff meeting in which George gleefully pointed out Rod's inferior monthly performance indicators and made inappropriate jokes suggesting that his cognitive abilities were declining with age, Rod finally sought assistance. As would be expected, Rod's emotional response was extremely muddled. He was clearly angry and embarrassed, but he was also sad that he was stuck in such an unpleasant work environment and somewhat scared that he might be in jeopardy of losing his job. Rod generated a number of possible responses ranging from trying to dig up dirt on George's personal character to blasting off a nasty, poisonous e-mail message and copying everyone in the company. When asked to consider his values in this situation, Rod was completely taken aback. Initially, he refused to look beyond George's behavior, but eventually when he opened to the possibility of exploring his personal values in the workplace he realized he had completely lost touch with what they actually were. With time, Rod was able to articulate his personal values of being direct and treating others fairly and with kindness. With a great deal of skepticism, but recognizing that he had few other options, Rod agreed to take some actions consistent with his values at work.

At the next staff meeting, George made his usual jab, trying to get a rise out of Rod, and Rod responded by making direct eye contact with him and thanking him for the feedback. George was so taken aback he was silent for the remainder of the meeting. Rod's manager pulled him aside and praised him for his calm behavior. Rod felt empowered and encouraged. As time went on, George recovered from his surprise and continued to needle Rod, but Rod used mindfulness practice and his values to guide his responses. He found that there were still some unpleasant moments at the office, but he was able to step back from his compulsion to control George and instead view him with some compassion. He was sorry that George couldn't escape the cycle of control attempts and focus on the things he cared about in his own life.

Our inability to control how other people act can be as frustrating as our inability to control our own internal experiences. And we can use the same skills to find a way to accept this reality. We can notice our reactions to others' actions, recognize our desires for things to be other than they are, and then choose the actions that are consistent with our own values. These actions may lead to a change in others' behavior, but they may not. Either way, we will know we are acting in ways that are meaningful to us. Often that alone can reduce our reactivity and distress in response to a specific context.

A metaphor drawn from Zen archery can be helpful here. When we shoot an arrow at a target, we can control how carefully we take aim, how far we draw back the bow, and precisely when we release the arrow. But other factors—a sudden gust of wind, for instance—will also influence where the arrow actually ends up. Our intentions as we prepare to shoot the arrow are appropriately focused on the outcome, on hitting the target, yet once we release the arrow we have to let go of outcome and let the arrow land where it lands. Similarly, we can do our best to choose our actions in ways that will contribute to optimal interactions with other people, yet at some point we have to realize that the outcome isn't only determined by us and let things be as they will be.

Everyone Has Values (Even If You Think You Don't)

Many people we work with have spent so much of their lives trying, unsuccessfully, to avoid experiencing anxiety and pain that they have lost any connection to what is important to them. Sometimes people feel that there isn't anything that truly matters to them, other than not being anxious. However, we always find that when people pay close attention and learn to let go of their habitual efforts to control and avoid their distress, they recognize what is important to them. As we described above, one way to find out what matters to you is to imagine what you would be doing if you did not experience anxiety, guilt, anger, or whatever distressing emotions you've been focusing on. Another option is to bring mindful awareness to your daily life and begin to notice the times that you experience satisfaction or a sense of meaning. This may happen in unexpected ways—when you have a particular type of interpersonal experience, when you solve a problem or fix something, or when you take some quiet time to yourself and reflect.

Sometimes people find they aren't sure what they value, or they feel torn between different options of what might be important. Often this reflects an indecisiveness that stems from a belief that there is a *correct* option. In fact, values are preferences, and no value is better than any other. It's like having a favorite ice cream or preferring Pepsi to Coke (or vice versa). There isn't a reason for the preference, and we don't have to explain to anyone why we like one ice cream flavor over another. What we value in relationships, work or school, and other areas of our lives has the same root—we value it because we prefer it and we find it satisfying and enriching. It may not be enriching to someone else, and it may not even always be enriching to us. But our values reflect our own sense of what is important and meaningful at a given time in our lives. So pay attention to your own inclinations and listen to them—don't feel like anyone else needs to agree with them. And be sure to use mindfulness so that you're listening to your preferences with an expanded, openhearted awareness, rather than a narrowed, reactive one.

Finding Value in Your Work

Often the domain of work/education/household management presents particular challenges as we try to identify what really matters to us. Some of us find our jobs inherently meaningful and can articulate why. Others, however, are ambivalent about our work or education— maybe we're not passionate about the job or academic course but chose it because we needed a job or an education. As with all values, there are no right or wrong answers to the question of what matters to you at work, but uncovering it can be tough. An important first step is asking the question "What matters to me here?" Bringing mindful awareness to a typical day as you go to school, care for your children, or go to work can help you identify the parts of these activities that feel meaningful and rewarding. Most likely you'll also notice aspects that don't feel rewarding.

If Values Are Not Morals, Can Harming or Taking Advantage of Others Be a Value?

Values and morals are not the same thing, but that does not mean that values aren't imbued with morals and ethics. In our experience, when people have been practicing mindfulness, allowing their emotional experiences, and cultivating compassion (discussed more fully in Chapter 12), actions that harm others hold little appeal. People certainly do engage in actions that hurt others all the time. However, these actions are typically driven by efforts to avoid one's own pain or the reality of a situation. When we allow ourselves to experience the full range of emotions and pay attention to everything that is occurring in the present moment, we are naturally drawn to actions that will not harm others. As we allow our own humanness and embrace it, we also see the humanness in others.

The "paddling out" metaphor introduced in Chapter 5 can be useful here. There may be aspects of your work or school that are dull or tedious or frustrating. Some of this "paddling out" may be necessary so that you can "ride the wave" from time to time and do what truly matters to you. For instance, reviewing 100 graduate student applications is an extremely tedious task that neither of us ever enjoys. However, mentoring a graduate student through her or his graduate experience is a highly valued action for both of us. We have to paddle through the applications if we want to ride this wave.

The trouble with our busy lives, however, is that we sometimes fail to notice that work or school or household management has become all paddling and no wave riding. The paddling can take up so much time and energy that we run out of steam and don't ever get to ride the wave, or don't even remember that riding the wave was the thing we loved. Bringing mindful awareness to our days can help us notice when the paddling takes so much time and energy that we never get to ride the wave or we've forgotten that the wave was what we loved about the work in the first place. With mindfulness practice we gain the ability to turn our attention back to the waves that brought us into this work or help us to find new waves if the old ones no longer appeal to us. Take

Daniel, who had a lucrative position as a sales manager in a large company, overseeing a team of salespeople.

Daniel initially felt good about being able to take care of his family financially, and he found many aspects of his job interesting and challenging. But gradually Daniel started to realize that he did not find the sales process inherently rewarding or its challenges exhilarating, as some of his coworkers did. Daniel began to judge himself critically for his career choice, and he became fused and entangled with his reactions. After reading an article about a corporate executive who quit his job, gave away his millions to charity, and joined the Peace Corps, Daniel began berating himself for having such a "useless" career. He experienced a gripping fear that his work had no meaning and that he was wasting his life. Soon he found himself begrudging his family the hours he put into his job to provide for them. As Daniel ruminated on the futility of his work, he became less motivated and more careless with his responsibilities. He began critically judging his coworkers as well and found himself engaging in battles with them. When his boss reprimanded him for the behavior, Daniel was fuming, and he told his wife he intended to quit his job, with or without another employment option. Daniel interpreted her fear and concern as selfish and invalidating, and conflict between the couple intensified. As Daniel's muddy emotions snowballed, his situation at work became more unpleasant and less fulfilling, setting off a vicious cycle of anxiety and despair.

In an attempt to respond differently to his anxiety, Daniel developed a mindfulness practice and began to bring openhearted awareness to his days. He noticed that he often had thoughts about his job not being meaningful and wishing he had a different job. He also noticed that he frequently reacted to these thoughts with judgment and self-criticism and that he vacillated between ruminating about them and trying to push them away. Daniel noticed that the behavior he engaged in when entangled in these thoughts was inconsistent with his values. He was irritable and short with coworkers, irresponsible and ineffective at work, and sharp with his family.

In addition to noticing, Daniel worked to bring compassion to his thoughts and emotions. He recognized that his dissatisfaction at work reflected his desire to contribute to humanity, which he came to identify as a core value. Daniel began exploring ways that he could take small actions consistent with these values through volunteerism and community action. Daniel also cultivated a compassionate stance toward himself as he considered the pressures and expectations society placed on him as a male "head of the household." As he brought mindfulness to his responses, Daniel was able to notice his thoughts arising and feel less fused to them, so that he was no longer chronically irritable. As his irritability subsided, he had more pleasant interactions with his coworkers. He then realized that he truly enjoyed managing and mentoring young sales associates and that he found that aspect of his work, which was a significant component of his job, extremely rewarding once he brought his attention to it. This realization led Daniel to find his work much more fulfilling, and he no longer felt resentful of his family.

Amelia was grateful that her partner's income made it possible for her to stay at home and take care of their three beautiful children. She could easily talk about what she valued about this work and the satisfaction she felt in caring for her children and keeping the house in order to make all of their lives better. Yet when she brought mindful awareness to her day, she noticed she often felt frustrated by the amount of work she had to do—the seemingly endless piles of laundry and dirty dishes, coordinating everyone's schedules, planning healthy meals that they could enjoy together in the midst of busy lives. When her partner came home from work and relaxed at the end of the day, Amelia was still at work, clearing the table, planning lunches for the next day, and helping the kids with their homework. In her daily routine, she had lost a connection to what she valued about what she was doing and rarely experienced the satisfaction she felt when she talked about her choice. This realization helped her bring more awareness to her daily routines and connect more intentionally to why she valued taking care of her family in this way. She was also able to ask her partner for assistance with

some tasks so that she could have time and energy for the relationship and self-nourishment domains of her life.

Many of us experience conflicts in our career choices, so that it can
seem difficult to choose a single path. Clark was in his senior year
of college, trying to decide what advanced degree to pursue. He
had always planned to pursue a law degree, confident that being
a lawyer would allow him to provide for his parents and siblings
financially, something that he valued a great deal. However, he
had found in the past year that he really enjoyed his African American studies courses, and he felt that a graduate degree in this area
would be extremely rewarding intellectually and would also allow
him to contribute more to his community as a whole. Clark faced a
choice that did not have a right answer—either option was clearly
a valued direction. After exploring the implications of both paths
and paying close attention to his own responses, Clark chose to
pursue law school. He asked his favorite African American studies
professor for suggestions of additional books he should read so that
he could continue to engage intellectually and emotionally with
this valued area of study and also decided that he would find some
volunteer work that was consistent with his values in this area. In
this way, he was able to honor both areas of importance, across the
domains of his life.

Jo had never thought much about work being meaningful. She felt
grateful for her job at the plant, because it helped keep a roof over
her family's head and put food on the table. She worked diligently
to make sure she would keep her job because she knew it would be
hard to get another one. But most of the time she was at work she
was waiting to get home to be with her friends and family. When
she brought awareness to her working day, she noticed how many
thoughts she had during the day about wanting to be elsewhere and
how those thoughts and the reactions she had to them made the day
drag on. She noticed that sometimes she had a moment of enjoying
the way her team worked together and felt good about her contri-

butions to the team output. She also noticed that when she was feeling frustrated with being at work, remembering that work was a way of providing for her family helped her not get entangled with those reactions. The reactions would still come, but they weren't as burdensome and her days didn't seem as never-ending. In this way, clarifying her values and bringing mindfulness to her experience helped Jo change her relationship with work even though her work remained the same.

You may face challenges similar to those faced by Daniel, Amelia, Clark, or Jo, or other complexities that we haven't represented here.

> *Sometimes experiencing an undercurrent of anxiety comes from not being able to find the meaning in your daily work.*

Bringing awareness to your day, noticing your clear and muddy emotions, and allowing yourself to explore what matters to you will help you find ways to work, study, and/or manage your household that are rewarding and meaningful, at least at times. Don't be discouraged if clarity about your values in this domain doesn't come easily or quickly. Just keep bringing openhearted awareness to your experience and see what you learn about how you might find value in the work you do.

EXERCISE **Clarifying your values in each domain**

Throughout this chapter you have explored what matters most to you. Now, as you prepare to move toward the life you want to live, it's helpful to review this exploration so you can zero in on a few areas in each of the three domains where you would like to make changes. Turn to a new page in your journal and write "Relationships" at the top. Then go back through all the writing you've done while reading this chapter to review what matters to you in relationships. Choose two or three things you value in your relationships that you would like to focus on for the next several weeks and write these on your page. Be sure to choose values that reflect your own sense of what is important, rather than someone else's, and that focus on actions rather than internal states you wish for. When your values relate to other people, focus on how you want to be in the relationship, including what you might want to ask of the other person. Now write "Work," "Education," or "Household

Management" at the top of another page (whichever is meaningful for you) and go through the same process, identifying two or three central values in this domain that you want to bring your awareness to. Finally, write "Self-Nourishment" and/or "Community Involvement" (if this is a value for you) at the top of another page and go through this process once more. Look back over what you've written, thinking about the discussion above, to be sure you've chosen values that reflect preferences rather than avoidance and that truly reflect what matters to you. If you find you are unsure about a value, that's OK. Write down your best guess of what is important to you in that domain. As you bring more awareness to this value and engage in actions mindfully, you will be able to discover whether you have accurately identified something that matters to you.

Before you read the next chapter, we would like you to take a week to monitor your value-guided actions (or valued actions, for short) in these domains. In your notebook, at the end of each day, write down any actions you took that were consistent with the ones you've identified. Also identify when there was an opportunity to take an action and you missed it. For instance, if one of your values is making connections with other people and someone asked you to lunch and you said no, this would be a missed opportunity. So write down the potential action and then write in a *T* if you took it and an *M* if you missed it. Also take note of how mindful you were (on a scale of 1 to 100) when you took or missed the opportunity to take an action. Finally, note any obstacles that got in the way of taking the action. These might be internal, such as feeling anxious or uncomfortable, or external, such as not being able to reach any of your friends when you called them on the phone. Becoming more aware of missed opportunities will be helpful over time, although you may find it discouraging at first. Remember to practice mindfulness with any distress you experience so you can accept your natural human responses and not let them interfere with the actions you've chosen based on your values. Continue your regular mindful practice throughout the week, using mindfulness of emotions (pages 131–132) or the clouds and sky mindfulness exercise (page 176) so that you continue to cultivate acceptance and willingness, which will help you continue to act in ways that reflect the values you've identified.

11

bringing it all together
MAKING A COMMITMENT TO YOURSELF

As we mentioned at the end of Chapter 6, it can be helpful to do a brief mindfulness practice before you read each chapter. If you haven't practiced yet, take a few moments now to do one of the formal practices you've been using regularly. This will help you fully engage in the material we discuss in this chapter and make the most of it. Try a practice that involves awareness of emotions or thoughts, like the clouds and sky mindfulness exercise or leaves on a stream from Chapter 9.

Now that you've begun to clarify what matters to you, and you've begun to learn to turn toward your internal experiences rather than habitually avoiding them, you're ready to put these two skills together and take direct steps to change your life. These changes may involve engaging in new actions, refraining from actions, or bringing more awareness to actions you've already been taking. As we discussed before, sometimes anxiety makes us a spectator in our lives so that even though we are living a full life, we aren't fully experiencing it. In these cases, bringing mindfulness to our actions may be the change we want to make. Before we talk about how to go about making these changes, it can help to think a bit about what it feels like to try to make changes in our lives.

Making a Commitment to Behavior Change

What thoughts or feelings arise when you think about making a commitment to changing your behavior? If you're like us, you may immediately find yourself thinking about all the reasons your efforts probably won't succeed. You may think about times when you tried to make changes in the past and failed. Or maybe you think you've been doing things the way you have for so long that you cannot even imagine another possibility. Or you may feel so excited about the idea of change that you want to implement all these changes immediately and find yourself feeling frustrated if change doesn't happen as quickly as you had hoped. It can be helpful to take some time to reflect mindfully on the reactions you have to the idea of committing to change.

EXERCISE **What does commitment mean to you?**

Please set aside 20 minutes to write about your responses to the idea of changing your behavior. As before, in your writing we want you to really let go and explore your very deepest emotions and thoughts about the topics listed below. It's important to allow yourself to experience your thoughts and feelings as completely as you can, because pushing these disturbing thoughts away can actually make them worse.

Write about any or all of the following topics, including just writing on one of the topics for 20 minutes. You may write about them in any order you wish. If you cannot think about what to write next, just write the same thing over and over until something new comes to you. Be sure to write for the entire 20 minutes. Please do not spend any time worrying about spelling, punctuation, or grammar—this writing is intended to be "stream of consciousness"—that is, you may write whatever comes to mind.

- What comes up for you when you think about making choices in your life and taking action based on what matters to you?

  — Do you often feel like your life is full of what you should do rather than what you want to do?

- — Are you doing what you want to do, but feeling disconnected from your actions?
- — Are there things you really want to do but feel unable to do because of your anxiety?
- What is the importance of the values you have chosen? What do they mean to you?
- What comes up for you when you think about the idea of willingness? What is the biggest obstacle that stands between you and the changes that you want to make?
- What negative and positive reactions come up for you when you think about making a commitment? What have been your past experiences in making commitments?

You may want to repeat this writing practice for several days in a row or later on, as you continue to think about making changes in your life and the obstacles that come up for you. This type of writing can help us connect to our motivations for making changes and also the fears that may keep us from engaging in valued actions. This awareness can help us more effectively move in directions that matter to us.

Common Responses to Efforts to Change Behavior

- "I won't succeed, so it's better if I don't even try."
- "I have too much going on to try to make any changes in my life right now."
- "I'm too anxious to make changes—I'll wait until I feel less stressed out."
- "I should be able to make these changes easily; if it takes so much effort there must be something wrong with me."
- "I've tried to make changes before and failed, so I should just give up."
- "Any time I fail in my efforts at changing my behavior, I should just give up."
- "I can't wait to get started—I wish these changes had already happened!"

All of us have had the experience of trying to make changes in our lives and not succeeding. Some of us may also have been successful in making some changes. It can be helpful to remember what has worked for us while we make plans to begin leading a more valued life. Sometimes the ideas we have about committing to change can be obstacles in and of themselves. Below we share some of our observations about making changes from our own experiences and from our work with other people.

Choice and Flexibility

Often we have gotten so used to reacting to situations and behaving automatically (e.g., avoiding anxiety-provoking situations, staying away from contexts that may cause us pain, trying to suppress our own distress) that it can take a while to get used to the idea of choosing our actions. Given your struggle with anxiety, chances are that, at least in some areas of your life, you tend to respond without thinking about it, without considering that you might actually have multiple options. This can happen for a few reasons. First, as described throughout the book, we often take our feelings as indications that we have to act in a certain way (avoid when we are anxious, shut down when we are sad, etc.). Second, our anxious behaviors can become strongly learned habits. For example, even if Sonia uses mindfulness to become more willing to experience the anxiety and self-critical thoughts that come up for her in social situations, she may find herself home alone in front of the television each night simply out of habit. You've begun to see that feelings and thoughts don't have to lead to actions as part of your mindfulness practice—you can feel like getting up, have the thought that your time could be better spent, or feel sensations that make you want to move your leg, yet you can keep practicing through that. Now we're going to work on applying that to the choices you make during your day.

An important part of living a value-guided life, then, is to recognize that our actions are choices, even if they don't feel like they are. At any moment we can ask ourselves, "Is this what I truly want to be doing in this moment?" As we begin to play our fourth round of a computer game instead of doing the work we had planned to do for the day, we can ask ourselves if this is the way we want to spend our time or if we want to make a different choice. This recognition that we can make choices is particularly important when we want to be living our lives in ways that may not be instantly gratifying but may lead to greater long-term satisfaction. Anyone who has ever tried to adhere to a healthier diet knows that it involves choosing not to eat what you feel like eating in the moment in the service of longer-term satisfaction. Or, if you want to meet someone special but don't *feel* like going on a first date, you'll have to do so if there's no one in your life right now whom you're interested in romantically.

Commitment Is an Intention, Not an Action

Have you ever decided to change your behavior and then gone against that decision and felt discouraged? So have we! One of the biggest challenges to making changes in our lives is figuring out how to respond to the inevitable "lapses" we'll experience as we go back on our commitments. No matter how strong our commitment, part of being human is recognizing that there are times when we'll act in ways that are inconsistent with our values, that we'll revert to anxious habits, and that we'll make mistakes. We find it helpful, therefore, to think of committing to change as an intention rather than an action. So we can be committed to getting into better physical shape, even as we decide not to go to the gym because we stayed up too late the night before. This allows us to keep our commitment so that we can try to engage in a consistent action the following day, rather than beating ourselves up so much that we give up altogether. This strategy was very helpful for me (L. R.) when I quit smoking. I never smoked a great quantity, but it had become a very ingrained habit in certain contexts and was very challenging to give up, even though I genuinely wanted to for my health. I found that each time I committed to quitting, I would face a situation in which I convinced myself that I could have "just one" and then I would feel discouraged later because I had "failed." This would lead me to stop trying to quit, and so I would continue smoking longer, feeling bad about myself for it. Finally I decided that I would make a clear commitment to quitting and that each time I lapsed I would have compassion for myself, because it was such a hard habit to break, and then I would recommit to quitting because I truly believed that it was better for me in the long run if I did not smoke. With this approach I was able to recover quickly each time I lapsed and return to my commitment to quit, and I eventually stopped smoking completely. Having compassion for myself in the process of quitting was also an important part of the process (see Chapter 12 for a more in-depth discussion of ways to cultivate self-compassion).

Smoking is a very concrete example, but there are many valued actions that are less concrete and yet equally (or more) challenging to make consistent changes in. Thinking of change as a process and commitment as an intention can help in these areas as well. Noushi valued being kind to her mother. However, her mother often said things that Noushi found hurtful, and she frequently reacted to these comments by saying something inconsiderate back to her mother. Afterward, Noushi would always feel bad and blame herself for not being kinder to her mother. As Noushi brought awareness to this pattern of interacting, she realized that blaming herself and feeling guilty was only muddying her emotions further and making it even more likely that she would snap at her mother, or even avoid talking to her altogether because the whole dynamic had become so unpleasant. When she brought compassion to herself for the responses she was having despite her best intentions, she found that her emotional responses became clearer and she was actually more able to respond kindly to her mother in most situations. There were still times that she slipped and said something petty or defensive, but when that happened she was more able to recover from it when she practiced mindfulness and recommitted to her intention to be kind to her mother.

As you've certainly noticed, it can be particularly challenging to take action in the face of anxiety. Carlos valued loyalty in his friendships and wanted to be someone who would stand up for a friend no matter what. However, in social situations his heart raced, his palms sweated, and his voice got shaky whenever he was the focus of attention. During lunch at work, one of his coworkers regularly insulted Carlos's friend. Carlos wanted to respond but could feel anxiety each time he started to say something, and so often he did not. Then he felt so bad about himself for letting his friend down that he became even more anxious and self-conscious. As Carlos brought gentle awareness to this situation, he was able to notice that he was automatically refraining from speaking because the anxiety symptoms were unpleasant. But he continued to feel uncomfortable nonetheless. So he made a commitment to acting in a way that was consistent with his values, regardless of the anxious sensations he experienced. He used his mindfulness skills to notice the sensations for what they were—normal bodily responses. And when his coworker began insulting his friend, he accepted those responses and spoke up anyway. He noticed the shaking in his voice and the anxious thoughts that arose about how others might see him. And he looked at his friend's face, connected to what mattered to him, and said something in support of his friend. Although he still felt uncomfortable when everyone looked at him, he also felt courageous and glad that he had spoken up.

EXERCISE **Mountain meditation**

The following exercise, from Jon Kabat-Zinn, is one of our favorites. It pulls together a lot of what you have been practicing up until now and cultivates an experience that can help you as you live the life you want to be living, while having all of the thoughts, feelings, and sensations that will inevitably arise. Set aside 15 minutes for this practice. As earlier, we use *-ing* words to impart a sense of the meditation being a process of continuing to bring awareness rather than of striving toward some end. You can download an audio recording of this exercise from the book website or read the description below before you practice it.

Pictur[ing] the most beautiful mountain you know or know of or can imagine, one whose form speaks personally to you. Focus[ing] on the image or the feeling of the mountain in your mind's eye, noticing its overall shape, the lofty peak, the base rooted in the rock of the earth's crust, the steep or gently sloping sides. Not[ing] as well how massive it is, how unmoving, how beautiful, whether seen from afar or up close ...

Perhaps your mountain has snow at the top and trees on the lower slopes. Perhaps it has one prominent peak, perhaps a series of peaks or a high plateau. However it appears, just sit[ting] and breath[ing] with the image of this mountain, observing it, noting its qualities. When you feel ready, see[ing] if you can bring the mountain into your own body so that your body sitting here and the mountain of the mind's eye become one. Your head becomes the lofty peak;

your shoulders and arms the sides of the mountain; your buttocks and legs the solid base rooted to your cushion on the floor or to your chair. Experienc[ing] in your body the sense of uplift, the ... elevated quality of the mountain deep in your own spine. Invit[ing] yourself to become a breathing mountain, unwavering in your stillness, completely what you are—beyond words and thought, a centered, rooted, unmoving presence.

Now, as well you know, throughout the day as the sun travels the sky, the mountain just sits. Light and shadow and colors are changing virtually moment to moment in the mountain's adamantine stillness. Even the untrained eye can see changes by the hour ... As the light changes, as night follows day and day night, the mountain just sits, simply being itself. It remains still as the seasons flow into one another and as the weather changes moment by moment and day by day. Calmness abiding all change.

In summer, there is no snow on the mountain, except perhaps for the very top or in crags shielded from direct sunlight. In the fall, the mountain may display a coat of brilliant fire colors; in winter, a blanket of snow and ice. In any season, it may at times find itself enshrouded in clouds or fog, or pelted by freezing rain. The tourists who come to visit may be disappointed if they can't see the mountain clearly, but it's all the same to the mountain—seen or unseen, in sun or clouds, broiling or frigid, it just sits, being itself. At times visited by violent storms, buffeted by snow and rain and winds of unthinkable magnitude, through it all the mountain sits. Spring comes, the birds sing in the trees once again, leaves return to the trees which lost them, flowers bloom in the high meadows and on the slopes, streams overflow with waters of melting snow. Through it all, the mountain continues to sit, unmoved by the weather, by what happens on the surface, by the world of appearances.

As we sit holding this image in our minds, we can embody the same unwavering stillness and rootedness in the face of everything that changes in our own lives over seconds, hours, and years. In our lives and in our [mindfulness] practice, we experience constantly the changing nature of mind and body and of the outer world. We experience periods of light and dark, vivid color and drab dullness. We experience storms of varying intensity and violence, in the outer world and in our own lives and minds. Buffeted by high winds, by cold and rain, we endure periods of darkness and pain as well as savoring moments of joy and uplift. Even our appearance changes constantly; just like the mountain's, it experiences a weather and a weathering of its own.

By becoming the mountain in [this exercise], we can link up with its strength and stability and adopt them for our own. We can use its energies to support our efforts to encounter each moment with mindfulness, equanimity, and clarity. It may help to see that our thoughts and feelings, our preoccupations, our emotional storms and crises, even the things that happen to us are more like the weather on the mountain. We tend to take it personally, but its strongest characteristic is impersonal. The weather of our own lives is not to be ignored or denied. It is to be encountered, honored, felt, known for what it is, and held in high awareness since it can kill us. In holding it this way, we come to know a deeper silence and stillness and wisdom than we may have thought possible, right within the storms. Mountains have this to teach us, and more, if we come to listen.

Value-Based Living

The mountain meditation may help us connect with our inner strength and stability and notice the transient nature of the thoughts and feelings that can seem to define us. Occasionally when we share this meditation with others, we hear concerns about how natural or human forces can erode a mountain. Sometimes people worry that their inner strength could also eventually be diminished by outside influences. It's true that, like mountains, we are clearly influenced by our environment and our outward appearance most definitely shifts and changes with time. But just as the mountain is more than its weather or outer appearance, our inner resources are stronger and more enduring than whatever passing thought, emotion, or physical sensation we might experience in a given moment.

We can bring the sense of strength and stability from the mountain (or whatever image or exercise helps us cultivate the sense of ourselves as distinct from our thoughts and feelings) to our intention to live a meaningful life. Now that you've identified what matters to you in each of the three domains and begun to bring your awareness to when opportunities to take value-based actions arise, you're ready to begin making commitments to valued action in your life. A good way to start making these changes is to choose an action or two you want to take each day, or several you would like to take in a week. It can be helpful to write these intentions down—you could use your notebook to write them down, perhaps one on a page, and then you can record whether you are able to act in a way that is consistent with your intention. If you do take a valued action, note whether you were able to be mindful during this action, and also anything that may have helped you to follow your intention. If you miss an intended action, note what obstacles got in your way and use that information to plan valued actions for the future.

> Oscar has been struggling with anxiety for years. He has realized that he has gradually narrowed his life more and more, in a futile effort to diminish his distress. He has begun practicing mindfulness and clarifying what matters to him and is now ready to begin to make changes in his life. He decides to begin by focusing on making connections with people (he feels isolated and misses interacting with other people) and improving his care of his physical health (his eating has been unhealthy, and he has stopped working out regularly for fear of having panic attacks). During his first day, he asks a coworker if she wants to grab lunch with him and suggests they go to a sandwich shop (instead of the fast-food place he usually frequents). Although he feels anxious making conversation during lunch, he also notices that it's nice to eat lunch with someone else and feels a sense of connection at moments. He acknowledges his anxiety as a message that he is taking risks, putting himself out there because he is a person who values having relationships in his life. When he has thoughts about how something he said sounded stupid, he notices them, brings some compassion to himself for having self-critical thoughts, and returns his attention to the conversation and the taste of his sandwich

At the end of the day, he has a number of thoughts about why he should stay late at the office to finish some work, briefly considers the messages he has received in his life about the priority of work in one's life, and chooses to go to the gym anyway. Although he notices his heart rate repeatedly while he runs on the treadmill, he remembers that the doctor said that his heart is healthy and that these are the kinds of reactions he always has to his heart rate, even when nothing is wrong. He is able to notice that it feels good to be running again, even as he continues to experience anxious thoughts. At the end of the day, Oscar feels pleased with himself for acting on his values so often during the day. It was challenging, and he felt uncomfortable at many points, yet he also feels the benefits of the choices he made.

Oscar had a particularly successful first day of value-guided action—we won't all have these, and Oscar's second day may not be quite as successful. But we can all learn from noticing how Oscar was able to engage in his valued actions. He continued to experience the same obstacles he has always experienced—he had distressing thoughts and physical sensations that were familiar to him. Rather than trying to get rid of these experiences, he *expanded* his awareness so that he was able to notice more positive experiences, like the feeling of running or the sense of connection at lunch, as well as the more distressing experiences that he habitually notices.

> *Anxiety narrows our attention, focusing it on what we find most threatening. Mindfulness expands our attention, helping us fully engage in our lives.*

Remember that anxiety naturally narrows our attention—the ability to mindfully expand awareness can help us have a more complete experience, noticing everything that is happening, rather than only what we find most threatening. Regularly practicing mindfulness helps Oscar in this situation—he is familiar with the kinds of anxious thoughts he has and knows that they will come and go, making it easier for him to expand his attention to the rest of his experience.

Oscar also used what he learned about the function of his emotion. In the past Oscar would have reacted to his anxiety with dread. He would have focused all of his attention on trying to calm down, and if his attempts failed he would have come up with an excuse to leave.

Instead, Oscar was able to acknowledge his emotion, accept its presence, and remain in the interaction.

When self-critical thoughts arose, rather than being carried off by a stampede of self-doubt, Oscar was able to observe them for what they were. He also brought compassion to his response, acknowledging for a moment how hard he is on himself and then returning his attention to the present moment.

Bringing Mindfulness to Current Valued Actions

The exercises in the previous chapter may have helped some of you realize that you already live a value-based life in many ways, but that you've become so preoccupied with worry and anxiety that you feel like a spectator in your own life. If this is the case, then engaging in valued action will mean bringing awareness to your current life so that you can enjoy the life you are already living. Informal mindfulness exercises can help you participate more fully in your life. The 3-minute breathing space, presented at the end of this chapter, is also an excellent practice to help with bringing awareness to our daily lives. Just before you engage in an action informed by what you value, take a few moments to practice so that you can bring heightened awareness to your action. And, as your mind wanders to other things, which it naturally will, notice it and bring it back to what you are doing right then so you can experience the satisfaction of doing what matters to you.

> *Mindfulness can help you stop being a spectator in your own life and start experiencing the satisfaction of doing what matters to you.*

Sometimes people find the practice of mindfulness so relaxing that they find themselves choosing to engage in formal practice instead of engaging in a valued life. Remember that participation in our lives is what we are working toward. Formal practice can definitely help us develop mindfulness skills that we can apply in our lives. But we can also find ourselves so drawn to the peace of our formal practice that we walk out of our lives to do it. Walking away to practice for 45 minutes is not the optimal way to resolve a tense discussion with your partner, for example. You may want to draw on your practice to notice your current reactivity, bring compassion to your experience, and remember your values in this context, but staying engaged with your partner will be an important part of any resolution.

Actions Can Be Big or Small

You may be wondering how to choose which actions to focus on to begin the process of living a life guided by what matters to you. You may feel like some of your values (e.g., being in an intimate, emotionally open relationship when you are currently single) are too large to address, while others (e.g., eating healthily) are too small to focus your energy on. In our experience, choosing a balance between more extensive values like ways of being in relationships, or finding satisfaction in work, and smaller, more concrete values that may be more readily addressed is optimal. In this way, you can enjoy the satisfaction of addressing more easily manageable valued actions that have been neglected and that can help you stay motivated to pursue changes in more challenging or complex areas. It can be tempting to leave the larger areas until later, but we find that, because these areas are often the ones that matter most, keeping them in mind and slowly making our way through changes in these areas is also helpful.

> Marisa went to therapy because she was experiencing extensive worry that was interfering with her life. She was dissatisfied with the level of emotional intimacy in her relationship with her boyfriend and concerned that she was not going to be able to have the type of relationship she valued with him. She also wanted to make changes in her community involvement. She had gone to church regularly growing up, but had not been able to find the time to become involved in a church since she had moved away from her family. She was hesitant to take on the value of emotional intimacy with her boyfriend, for fear it would "make things worse" and lead to their breakup. Yet she felt like community involvement really was not a priority in her life at the moment and so was also reluctant to approach this area. As she and her therapist explored her values in each area, it became clear that she was not living according to her values in either domain, and Marisa could see that this was having a negative effect on her life. Her therapist suggested that she attend to both areas in the coming week, and he and Marisa explored

ways she might address each value. Marisa decided that she would make a list of potential churches in her area and attend one that Sunday to see what she thought of it. She also decided to share her emotional experience with her boyfriend at least once during the week, to see whether one of the obstacles to their intimacy was her reluctance to be emotionally vulnerable.

Marisa and her therapist found a way to take a meaningful step in a large area in her life (emotional intimacy with her boyfriend) at the same time that she took a significant step in a smaller yet important area in her life. By addressing both areas at once, Marisa can see what it feels like to move toward things she has been avoiding in different contexts and has a better chance of finding some success and satisfaction from her initial efforts.

> *Taking both large and small actions can help you experience success in moving toward what you've been avoiding in different contexts.*

We can also identify small steps in big areas of our lives and start with those. Erik wanted to be in an intimate relationship, but he experienced so much social anxiety that he completely avoided talking to new people. The idea of pursuing dating seemed impossible to him and clearly wasn't going to be a good place for him to start. Instead, he was able to identify initial actions, like saying hello to someone in the elevator or asking someone for her notes after class, that elicited a great deal of anxiety and discomfort that he could be willing to experience. Engaging in these actions was an important step toward making new connections, which was consistent with his value of cultivating an intimate relationship. As he engaged in more of these actions, his anxiety diminished a bit and he found that he actually enjoyed conversations with new people, even though they elicited anxiety. This new learning helped him make the next step and begin online dating.

Addressing Obstacles

As you bring awareness to the choices you are making and commit to taking valued actions in specific areas of your life, you will undoubtedly find that a number of apparent obstacles arise. Some will be internal obstacles and some external. Internal obstacles are any thoughts, feelings, or sensations that lead us to feel we cannot do something. You've seen that these obstacles can be addressed by cultivating willingness. Your mindfulness practice, understanding of the function of emotion, willingness to let go of the struggle with control, and growing ability to see thoughts as thoughts, rather than statements of truth, will help you continue to engage in the action that matters to you while having whatever responses you have, as Oscar did.

Internal obstacles begin to seem more challenging when emotions are muddy. Chapter 7 described numerous ways that emotions can go from clear to muddy, making them more intense and more difficult to understand. When you find that your emotional responses present an obstacle to your valued actions, ask yourself whether your emotions are muddy. If they are, bring mindfulness to your emotions. You may want to use the mindfulness of emotions exercise in Chapter 6, or "inviting a difficulty in" in Chapter 12 to help you turn toward your experience and open up to your distress, so that it can become less muddy and more clear. These practices will make it easier for you to choose to act in ways that matter to you, regardless of your internal state.

As you try to make changes so you can live in ways that matter to you, you'll probably also encounter external obstacles. Maybe you want to be more social, but you work at home, so you never meet anyone new. Or you may want to feel challenged in your work, but you feel like you've mastered your current job. Problem solving can help you come up with alternatives that will allow you to pursue the actions that matter to you. Don't be afraid to ask others for suggestions when you feel stuck.

Remember that it will be natural to rule out some of the alternatives you come up with because they may elicit discomfort or anxiety. However, living a value-guided life means moving toward what matters to you

> *Living a value-based life means moving toward what matters to you rather than away from what provokes anxiety—so consider even the solutions that make you uncomfortable when trying to remove obstacles.*

rather than away from anxiety-provoking things. So, although online dating may sound unpleasant, it may be a wonderful way to open yourself up to new people. Similarly, joining a club or getting involved in an activity may be a good way to open up your social circle. And, although it may be uncomfortable to ask a boss for new assignments, you can still do it if that challenge at work matters to you. If you've found external obstacles to some of the valued actions you've identified, take some time now to brainstorm potential avenues for moving forward in these valued directions and write them down in your journal. Write down anything that comes to mind, no matter how bizarre it sounds. Then you can review your list and choose which you want to try first.

Is Your Anger Clear or Muddy?

As we discussed in Chapter 7, distinguishing between clear and muddy emotions is an important part of living a full and meaningful life. Clear emotions give us information that may guide our actions, while muddy emotions tell us that we are having reactions to our emotions due to poor self-care, worrying or ruminating, judgments of our experience, or efforts to control our responses. Mindfulness exercises can help us clarify our muddy emotions or at least recognize the muddiness so that we know not to listen to what our emotions are screaming at us.

Distinguishing between clear and muddy emotions can be challenging, though, and there are no set rules about which emotions tend to be clear versus muddy, although you may begin to find that certain emotions are often muddy for you while others are more likely to be clear. Anger is a good example of this variability. People have very different relationships to this emotion and are often socialized very differently about anger. Some of this varies by gender, although people of both genders can have a range of responses to anger. Often men have learned that anger is one of the few acceptable emotions. As a result, when they experience more vulnerable emotions, like fear or sadness, they quickly respond with anger. This leads them to feel less vulnerable, but it interferes with their ability to learn what their initial emotion was communicating to them. In this case, anger is a muddy emotion because it occurs in response to an initial clear emotion. If you find that you are often angry or agitated, it may be that anger is commonly a muddy emotion for you and that by turning toward it and practicing mindfulness exercises (like mindfulness of emotions in Chapter 6, mindfulness of emotions and physical sensations in Chapter 7, clouds and sky mindfulness in Chapter 9, or inviting a difficulty in, in Chapter 12), you may be able to find the clear emotion underneath it.

On the other hand, women are often socialized not to express their anger and to turn away from it. As a result, they often experience anxiety, guilt, or shame in response to any inkling of anger. In this case, anger is a clear emotion that may be communicating that someone's rights have been violated. However, the muddy emotional response interferes with this important message, making it difficult to take actions to correct the situation. If you find that you are rarely angry but often experience anxiety, guilt, or shame, you may find that turning toward these experiences and practicing the exercises listed above may help you identify any clear emotions of anger that may provide useful information. Of course, some men are socialized not to express or experience anger, and some women are encouraged to express anger rather than more vulnerable emotions. It can be helpful to think of your own relationship to anger and to use that as you try to sort through your clear and muddy emotions.

Finding Balance

You may find that as you turn your attention toward one valued domain (e.g., relationships), another suffers (e.g., work). In our experience, some degree of imbalance is unavoidable. There are times in our lives when we may focus a great deal on school or work and some of the other areas of our lives may suffer. Or we may have certain days of the week when our responsibilities in one domain make it difficult to attend to any others. Nonetheless, bringing our awareness to all three areas can help us make sure that we maintain some balance over time. Otherwise, some areas (like self-care or community involvement) may be so habitually neglected that we find over time that we are not living in accordance with our values in these domains at all. We are more likely to feel satisfied in our lives if we attend to each area at some point so that we have some balance overall, even if not in a given day or week. By clarifying our values in all domains and reminding ourselves of the full range of what matters to us, we are more likely to respond flexibly in a given moment to maintain balance.

For instance, I (L. R.) am currently very focused on writing this chapter because we promised our editor we would give her a full draft of the manuscript soon. This is consistent with my value of using what we have learned over the years in our research and clinical work to help as many people as possible. In prioritizing this value over the past several days, I have set aside long periods of time to write and edit and plan for the book. My partner has very graciously picked up many household chores to help me pursue my value in my work domain.

However, today when I was walking home from a quick errand, very focused on what I would write next once I got inside and to my computer, I noticed that our sidewalk needed to be shoveled *again* (the joys of January in New England). I immediately had the thought that my partner would do it, as I prepared to run upstairs and resume my position in front of the computer. Then I remembered that he'd already spent several hours shoveling in the past few days. And I thought about how I value sharing the responsibilities of maintaining our home, even though my partner often takes on more of these responsibilities because my work takes up so much time. And I noticed how automatically I had assumed that I couldn't possibly do this now, because I had to write. I took a breath, reflected on the choice I wanted to make, and reached for a shovel.

Over the next 45 minutes, I had a number of thoughts about how cold and wet I was, how much I needed to write, and how I wished our neighbors were helping with the shoveling. At the same time, I also felt satisfaction as I cleared our sidewalk so that no one would slip and fall. And while my arms started to hurt a bit, I noticed that it was nice to get a little bit of an upper-body workout after sitting at the computer for so long. And I felt satisfaction knowing that my partner would at least get a break from shoveling this one day. And, when a teenage girl walked by on the phone saying, "Don't cry over him. Stop crying," I was happy for the reminder of why I wanted to get back to writing about ways to turn toward our feelings instead of away from them and live a fuller life.

This small example also illustrates the way our valued actions are a choice and that there are no right or wrong answers. I certainly could have chosen to go inside and write instead of shoveling (and my editor may think that would have been the right choice!). Sometimes, we have to choose between two equally valued options, and those choices are never easy. Yet if we are aware and intentional, we can be sure to balance out these choices over time. Today, having chosen work over contributing to our household management for so many days in a row, I chose shoveling. On another day I might choose writing. The key is to remember that these are choices and to pay attention to the consequences of our choices.

Process Rather Than Outcome

As we discussed in the last chapter, living a value-based life is a process, not something that we achieve and then are done with. It can be helpful to begin this process by choosing specific actions for a day or a week and seeing how that turns out and then choosing more actions. But eventually we want to respond more flexibly, noticing in a given moment what matters to us and acting accordingly.

Often, people who have experienced a lot of anxiety in their lives have developed a habit of trying to do things very well or perfectly all the time. While this habit can serve people very well and lead to a lot of success in different areas, it can also lead to a lot of distress and continued anxiety and get in the way of living a full, valued life. If this describes you, you may find that as you begin to engage in valued actions you are often frustrated that you are not fully living in accordance with your values or that you cannot live in a valued way in all domains at once. The next chapter helps you cultivate self-compassion, which will allow you to keep moving in valued directions, despite setbacks and obstacles, without getting frustrated for not being perfect.

> *Perfectionism is a side effect of anxiety that can be avoided if you think of valued actions as a process rather than an end in themselves.*

Instead of aiming for perfection in our valued actions, we find it helpful to think of these actions as moving in a direction. At any given moment I can choose to be more open-hearted, caring, diligent, truthful, creative, or whatever else I value. That doesn't mean that I will necessarily be as creative as I could possibly be (in fact, the more I want that, the more elusive it is likely to be). Yet I can find satisfaction in the experience of moving in the direction of what is important to me and recognize that progress. As you continue identifying and pursuing actions based on your values, see if you can keep this idea of movement in a valued direction in mind and see whether that helps you move forward.

Values clarification is also a process. As you begin engaging in actions that matter to you and finding more flexibility in your life, you may begin to wonder whether the values you have identified truly reflect what is most important to you. This is very natural. If these questions arise, you may want to write about your values again, to explore the new ideas that are arising for you. In general, we recommend sticking to a specific valued action for a couple of weeks before you give it up, so that you can see whether these questions arise from avoidance or impatience (both very human responses, particularly because the process of change can be so slow) or reflect new awareness on your part. The best way to determine whether we truly value something is to try out acting consistent with that value and see if it leads to more satisfaction in our lives. Remember that satisfaction does not mean minimal distress—instead, we are referring to a deeper sense of fulfillment and meaning, which can co-occur with distress. This is the feeling we all get when we are living a life that truly matters to us.

Remembering to Take Valued Action

We all tend to go through our days habitually, so it's easy not to notice opportunities to practice valued action or bring mindfulness to our actions. Making a commitment at the beginning of the day can help to bring our values into our minds. Another helpful tool is practicing mindfulness during our day. Informal practice (such as washing dishes mindfully, riding the elevator mindfully, bringing awareness to our breath before we answer the phone) is one way of enhancing mindfulness throughout the day. Take a few moments to think of a few informal practices that you want to bring into your day and write them in your notebook. See how the feeling of your day changes as you regularly bring mindfulness to your daily life.

EXERCISE **Three-minute breathing space**

This is a briefer exercise, developed by Zindel Segal and his colleagues, that puts together a lot of what we've been practicing over longer periods. This will allow you to use this kind of practice during your day, giving you another way to apply mindfulness to your life, in addition to practicing it more formally as you have been. The exercise is designed to be like an hourglass—first you'll bring awareness to your experience (the top wide part), then you'll narrow to your breath, to ground you, then you'll expand back out.

The first thing to do is to take a very definite posture ... relaxed, dignified, back erect, but not stiff, letting your body express a sense of being present and awake.

Now, closing your eyes, if that feels comfortable for you, the first step is being aware of what is going through your mind. What thoughts are around? Here, again, as best you can, just noting the thoughts as mental events ... So we note them, and then noting the feelings that are around at the moment ... in particular, turning toward any sense of discomfort or unpleasant feelings. So rather than trying to push them away or shutting them out, just acknowledging them, perhaps saying, "Ah, there you are, that's how it is right now." And similarly with sensations in the body ... Are there sensations of tension, of holding, or whatever? And again, awareness of them, simply noting them. OK, that's how it is right now.

So you've got a sense of what is going on right now. You've stepped out of automatic pilot. The second step is to collect your awareness by focusing on a single object—the movements of the breath. So focusing attention down there in the movements of the abdomen, the rise and fall of the breath ... spending a minute or so focusing on the movement of the abdominal wall ... moment by moment, breath by breath, as best you can. So that you know when the breath is moving in, and you know when the breath is moving out. Just binding your awareness to the pattern of movement down there ... gathering yourself, using the anchor of the breath to really be in the present.

And now as a third step, having gathered yourself to some extent, allowing your awareness to expand. As well as being aware of the breath, also including a sense of the body as a whole. So that you get this more spacious awareness ...

A sense of the body as a whole, including any tightness or sensations related to holding in the shoulders, neck, back, or face ... following the breath as if your whole body is breathing. Holding it all in this slightly softer ... more spacious awareness.

And then, when you are ready, just allowing your eyes to open.

You may have found the 3-minute breathing space to be surprisingly brief and may find that you miss the effects of longer practice. Nonetheless, this can be a very useful way to cultivate mindfulness in the midst of a busy day. Use this exercise when you find yourself feeling overwhelmed or like you've lost track of what is important to you in a given moment. You also may find it helpful just before you engage in a valued action, as a way of increasing your mindfulness so that you can bring it into the meaningful context, like a conversation with a loved one, or an important meeting at work.

Another important practice to maintain your commitment to value-guided action is bringing your awareness back to your values and what matters to you. Because valued action so often involves engaging in something that may not feel good in the moment, but that we expect to be meaningful in the long run, being connected to the reason that we do something can help us carry out our chosen action. Getting in the habit of reviewing your notebook or doing writing assignments from time to time can help you stay connected to what really matters to you so that this can guide your actions.

Guidelines for Engaging in Actions Based on Your Values

- Bring awareness to the way you are feeling.
  - Are your feelings clear or muddy?
  - Practice mindfulness (of emotions, physical sensations and

emotions, clouds and sky, inviting a difficulty in) to clarify emotions.

— What information do your clear emotions give you about what matters to you in this context?

- Are you trying to control or avoid your internal experience?

  — Cultivate mindfulness and willingness.

  — Remind yourself what matters to you in this domain.

- Cultivate compassion for yourself.

- Bring awareness to what matters to you and use that to motivate your actions.

- Participate fully, mindfully in your chosen actions.

- Regularly review all three domains to be sure you are engaging in valued actions across domains and across time.

- When you fail to take valued actions, cultivate self-compassion, explore the obstacles and address them, and recommit to your chosen actions.

12

overcoming challenges
to cultivating self-compassion

As you have undoubtedly noticed, cultivating a mindful stance requires both patience and practice. The mind naturally wanders, and becoming more aware of its meandering as well as learning to escort your attention back to the present moment can take considerable effort. Observing or moving toward anxiety is also an adjustment, particularly since our usual mode is to turn away from anxious thoughts, emotions, bodily sensations, and images. The mind often resists beginner's mind as it is constantly seeking shortcuts or quicker ways to process information. Yet we hope you have also noticed the benefits of mindfulness: the occasional quieting of the mind ... the deeper connections you can forge with loved ones and friends ... how becoming aware of anxiety earlier in the cycle helps us catch habitual responses like judgment and control efforts that only fan the flames of anxiety. Although repeated practice can ease the challenges of mindfulness, recall that mindfulness is a process and not a final state that can be achieved. Even the most experienced teachers and Buddhist priests need to regularly practice applying mindfulness skills in response to the natural inclination of their minds to wander, self-criticize, and judge.

One of the most challenging skills of mindfulness to incorporate into daily life is self-compassion. Psychologist Kristen Neff describes self-compassion as "being open to and moved by one's own suffering,

237

experiencing feelings of caring and kindness toward oneself, taking an understanding, nonjudgmental attitude toward one's inadequacies and failures, and recognizing that one's experience is part of the common human experience" (p. 224). When we are self-compassionate, we recognize that part of being human is making mistakes and experiencing difficulties. We see our experiences and struggles as reflective of the human condition, rather than as personal shortcomings. Instead of hiding our imperfections, or engaging in harsh self-criticism, we gently allow ourselves to acknowledge and learn from our experiences. This self-orientation can buffer us against life's difficulties and enhance our emotional resilience.

EXERCISE **Reflections on self-compassion**

In the monitoring exercises, we asked you to notice when you were judgmental and self-critical, and we suggested that you practice bringing self-compassion to your anxious responses. Self-compassion is also a skill we asked you to practice through the mindfulness exercises. Have you been able to bring self-compassion to these experiences? If so, what has that experience been like for you? If you have struggled with bringing compassion to your experience, what has been getting in the way? When you think about self-compassion, do any concerns arise? Do you have any thoughts about the origin of those concerns? Do you find it easier to be self-critical than to be compassionate toward yourself?

Obstacles to Self-Compassion

Practice can make compassion, like the other skills of mindfulness, more habitual. But because we all have such a strong inclination to judge many of our internal responses critically and harshly, you might find you encounter roadblocks. Anxiety is often associated with habitual self-criticism, which interferes with self-compassion. In this chapter we consider the obstacles that may stand in your way of cultivating self-compassion and introduce some exercises aimed at enhancing this elusive but valuable component of mindfulness practice.

Viewing Emotional Responses as Unacceptable

Sometimes people struggle with self-compassion because they judge their emotional responses to be unacceptable. In Chapter 6, we discussed the central role emotions play in our lives. Emotions are universal, extremely informative, and help us adapt to the challenges of daily life. Yet they are not always honored and valued. Social and cultural norms can dictate whether the expression of emotion is appreciated or devalued. As we described in Chapter 8, emotional experiences, such as fear, sadness, or anger, can be viewed as signs of weakness or a lack of self-control, so that they often automatically elicit self-criticism and judgment, which are the opposite of self-compassion. These judgments can become such a habit for us that we don't even notice the harsh responses we continually have to our own emotional reactions. Furthermore, our own confusion about emotions when they are muddied by poor self-care, thoughts about the future, memories of past events, fusion, and/or critical reactions can lead us to become even more judgmental and nonaccepting. This judgment and self-criticism can lead to even more muddy emotions, which are judged even more harshly, creating a cycle of distress. Becoming aware of the function of our emotions, understanding the ways they can become muddied, and bringing clarity to our responses when they arise can help increase our compassion. In addition, bringing self-compassion to any emotional experience we have, regardless of how muddy or intense it is in the moment, can stop the cycle of escalating distress and anxiety and help to clarify our emotional responses.

Bringing compassion to our emotional responses can be extremely challenging, particularly when we've learned to respond the opposite way to these feelings. The poem "The Guest House" (at the beginning of Chapter 9) seems so foreign when we first encounter it because building a barrier to emotions, rather than inviting them in, is such a common, habitual response. Yet this response leads to constriction in our lives, rather than willingness and freedom. Cultivating mindfulness toward these emotional responses is therefore a very important part of learning to live a value-guided life. We and the people with whom we've worked have found the following mindfulness exercise, adapted from *The Mindful Way through Depression*, particularly helpful in cultivating self-compassion. This exercise uses the physical sensations that arise in the presence of challenging emotions to help us learn to respond to these emotions with gentleness and care instead of judgment.

EXERCISE **Inviting a difficulty in and working with it through the body**

Before you begin this exercise, think of a difficulty you're experiencing right now. It doesn't have to be a significant difficulty, but choose something that you find unpleasant, something that is unresolved. It may be something you are worried about, an argument or misunderstanding you've had, something you feel angry, resentful, guilty, or frustrated about. If nothing is going on right now, think of some time in the recent past when you felt scared, worried, frustrated, resentful, angry, or guilty, and use that. Now read through the following script and then practice this exercise, sitting on a cushion or a chair. You can also download a recording of the exercise from the book website. (Again, we've used the *-ing* form of verbs to give the sense of mindfulness as a process, not a destination.)

Noticing the way you are sitting in the chair or on the floor. Noticing where your body is touching the chair or floor. Bringing your attention to your breath for a moment. Noticing the in breath ... and the out breath ... Now gently widening your awareness, take in the body as a whole. Noticing any sensations that arise, breathing with your whole body.

When you are ready, bringing to mind whatever situation has been bringing up difficult emotions for you. Bringing your attention to the specific emotions that arise and any reactions you have to those emotions. And as you are focusing on this troubling situation and your emotional reaction, allowing yourself to tune in to any *physical sensations* in the body that you notice are arising ... becoming aware of those physical sensations ... and then deliberately, but gently, directing your focus of attention to the region of the body where the sensations are the strongest in the gesture of an embrace, a welcoming ... noticing that this is how it is right now ... and *breathing into that part of the body* on the in breath and breathing out from that region on the out breath, exploring the sensations, watching their intensity shift up and down from one moment to the next.

Now, seeing if you can bring to this attention an even deeper attitude of compassion and openness to whatever sensations, thoughts, or emotions you are experiencing, however unpleasant, by saying to yourself from time to time, "It's OK. Whatever it is, it's already here. Let me open to it."

Staying with the awareness of these internal sensations, breathing with them, accepting them, letting them be, and allowing them to be just as they are. Saying to yourself again, if you find it helpful, "It's here right now. Whatever it is, it's already here. Let me be open to it." Softening and opening to the sensation you become aware of, letting go of any tensing and bracing. If you like, you can also experiment with holding in awareness both the sensations of the body and the feeling of the breath moving in and out as you breathe with the sensations moment by moment.

And when you notice that the bodily sensations are no longer pulling your attention to the same degree, simply return 100% to the breath and continue with that as the primary object of attention. And then gently bringing your awareness to the way you are sitting in the chair, your breath, and, when you are ready, opening your eyes.

Pia had an argument with her teenage daughter, Leah, before school in the morning. Leah arrived at the kitchen table wearing a skimpy tank top and ripped jeans. Pia reminded her that these were her weekend clothes, not clothes she was allowed to wear to school. Leah responded with anger and ended their argument by storming out of the room, shouting, "I hate you! You don't care about me!" On her way to her therapy appointment, Pia kept replaying the exchange, feeling anxious, with sensations of tightness in her chest and stomach as she recalled the look of anger on Leah's face. She found herself worrying about Leah's recent moodiness and rebellion and imagining that the conflict in their relationship was going

to just worsen. Pia kept telling herself to let it go, not to worry, not to let Leah get to her that way. But her mind returned to the image again and again, as she obsessed about the future of their relationship. She told her therapist about what had happened and agreed to practice "inviting a difficulty in" to work with her emotional responses. After spending several minutes breathing into her chest and belly, opening up to the physical sensations of anxiety, the tightness and pain she felt, Pia felt the tightness release, and tears came to her eyes. She felt deep sadness at the emotional distance between her daughter and her. She also felt profound love for Leah and concern for her well-being. As she repeated to herself, "It's already here," she felt how this pain and struggle were an integral part of loving this human being through this stage of development. When she opened her eyes, she felt at peace with the sadness and the fears of parenting a teenager, and remembered as well the joys that came from this experience. She felt compassion for herself and also for Leah, as they made their way, together and apart, through this challenging time.

Often when we open up to our emotional experiences and allow them, we can really feel how they are a part of our humanness and a part of living a full, meaningful life. This exercise is a helpful way of accessing this experience. Many people we have worked with have found, over time, that simply repeating the phrase "It's OK; it's already here" can help them drop their struggle with their emotions and open up their feelings of self-compassion. Use this exercise in your own life when you feel like you are fighting with your anxiety or other emotions or criticizing yourself for having them and see what emerges when you soften toward your experience instead of trying to keep it at bay.

Believing Self-Compassion Means Heaping False Praise on Ourselves

Some resistance to the idea of self-compassion springs from a misunderstanding of the concept. For example, one may equate self-compassion with the loosely related, but distinct, concept of self-esteem. Self-esteem refers to a self-evaluation or judgment about how much we like, appreciate, or value ourselves, often relative to other people. Although it is a widely popular concept in our society and many initiatives and efforts are aimed at increasing self-esteem, there has also been some backlash and controversy surrounding the concept. At first glance, it seems difficult to argue against the benefits of helping people feel positive about themselves or special. The trouble with self-esteem is that it is often anchored to performance, achievement, or appearance. If I make the elite baseball team, acquire a fancy sports car, or have a pleasing physical appearance, I may have high self-esteem. But if I end up on the bench, drive a clunker, and put on some weight, my self-esteem may plummet. The movement away from competitive contests in schools and sports was motivated by the belief that coming in last place in the school spelling bee or being the slowest in a race might harm a developing child's self-esteem. On the other hand, some have argued that these practices lead to falsely inflated perceptions of abilities and intolerance of struggle or failure. In other words, if Daniel is praised lavishly for his performance whether or not he exerts any real effort or has any skill, in the service of increasing his self-esteem, he may develop real behavioral and interpersonal problems. Many argue that high self-esteem is necessary for a happy and successful life, but the research on self-esteem produces mixed findings. It seems like moderately high self-esteem may be associated with well-being, but high self-esteem has also been connected with self-absorption, narcissism, and problems with social functioning.

In contrast, self-compassion is an unwavering stance we hold toward ourselves that is independent of achievement, appearance, or behavior. It doesn't require self-evaluation, | *Self-compassion does not equal self-esteem.* |

self-comparison, or judgment. This stance can be maintained through successes, failures, praise, and blame. Furthermore, the compassion we generate for ourselves comes from the recognition that all humans are imperfect and everyone experiences suffering. The assumption is that not only do we have compassion for ourselves; we also have compassion for all humans as they face similar struggles.

Believing Self-Compassion Means Ignoring or Denying Our Mistakes

Some people fear that self-compassion requires sugarcoating reality or seeing one's behavior through rose-colored glasses. Interestingly, psychologist Mark Leary recently found that people high in self-compassion are actually more accurate in their observation and evaluation of their own behavior than those low in self-compassion. He and his colleagues also found that when people are self-compassionate they are more likely to take personal responsibility for a negative event and less likely to be overwhelmed by distress resulting from the event. Similarly, psychologist Kristen Neff found that students high in self-compassion were more likely to consider receiving an unsatisfactory grade on a midterm to be an opportunity for growth and improvement and less likely to focus on negative feelings or use avoidance as a coping strategy. Students high in self-compassion were

> *Taking a self-compassionate stance means accepting your inherent worth.*

also unique in that they were academically motivated more by curiosity and the desire to develop skills than by the need to defend or enhance feelings of self-worth.

Fearing Self-Compassion Will Turn You into a Lazy Softie

Some people worry that if they are self-compassionate they will lose their motivation to work hard and "do the right thing" and instead will become lazy and complacent. This reaction reflects a deeply ingrained cultural belief that punishment enhances motivation. Brian was a client we saw in therapy who strongly objected to the idea that he should bring self-compassion to his fear and anxiety. He thought increased self-discipline and a steely resolve to face his fears were what he needed to advance in treatment. Brian drew an analogy between the tough, "no-excuses" philosophy he brought to his anxiety and his strict authoritarian approach to parenting. Brian frequently expressed his viewpoint that children these days suffered from a lack of self-discipline that put them at risk for behavioral problems and underachievement. He attributed this growing problem to a cultural shift toward permissive parenting and parents' unwillingness to assert their authority and punish their children for inappropriate behavior.

Similarly, Brian believed the lack of self-discipline and a general "softening" of our society was contributing to the rising prevalence of anxiety and depression. Brian believed that his own battle with anxiety could be overcome with mental toughness. But given his lack of success in applying these principles to his own behavior, he skeptically expressed a willingness to consider another approach.

Despite Brian's firm belief in the benefits of his authoritarian style of parenting, he admitted that he had a rocky relationship with his children and wished they were closer. He also conceded that his children regularly misbehaved and got into trouble despite his unwavering commitment to household rules and his consistent follow-through with punishment. Brian's take on the situation was that his anxiety made him appear weak and that it was undermining his parental authority. Initially he clung to the belief that he needed to come down harder on himself and his children, but as Brian's frustration and hopelessness grew, he agreed to consider other explanations and solutions.

Brian was becoming more observant and aware of his own behavior and its associated consequences through mindfulness practice. Thus we invited him to use these skills to objectively evaluate the accuracy of some of his core beliefs about parenting. After a few weeks of careful self-monitoring, Brian discovered that while many punishments and restrictions had the desired short-term effect, there appeared to be subtle, unintended longer-term adverse consequences. Brian's children rarely disagreed with him or questioned his authority when he attempted to restrict or control their behavior at home, but they repeatedly acted out at school and in unsupervised situations. Brian noticed that his children did not seem to internalize the lessons he was trying to impart. Although they would "talk the talk" in his presence, dutifully using polite language and completing their chores, behind his back they often cheated, lied, and behaved aggressively. Like many children raised by authoritarian parents, Brian's children were resentful about the punishment and restrictions on their behavior and showed little motivation to act in ways consistent with his values when they were freed from his control. Paradoxically, the more harsh and critical Brian was in response to his children's behavior, the more trouble they caused.

Although initially skeptical about alternative parenting styles, Brian acknowledged that his methods seemed to be ineffective and that they might be poisoning his relationship with the children. We shared with Brian the wealth of evidence from both animal and learning research that rewarding positive behavior is more effective than punishing negative behavior. After a few weeks of "catching his children being good" and reinforcing them for positive actions, Brian was impressed with the modest but significant improvement in their behavior and the impact on the harmony within his home.

We then asked Brian to bring the same beginner's mind and careful observation to the consequences of self-criticism on his emotional state and behavior. We asked him to observe the relationship between threats and harsh self-criticism and motivation and follow-through. After a few weeks of self-monitoring, Brian saw a similar pattern emerge. Although self-threats seemed to motivate his behavior in the short term, they backfired in the long term. For instance, Brian used negative self-talk such as "You are fat, lazy, and ugly, and Debbie is going to divorce you unless you work out and lose 50 pounds by the summer" to motivate himself to get out

> *Self-criticism is only a short-term motivator.*

of bed and go to the gym after a sleepless, anxiety-ridden night. These harsh threats propelled him to the gym 3 days in a row, but by day 4 he was disgusted and ready to quit. Brian couldn't think about exercise without hearing judgments and criticisms, and the thoughts generated considerable sadness, anger, and hopelessness. Overwhelmed by muddy thoughts and emotions, he turned to distraction as a method of self-soothing and preserving his sense of self-worth. Brian started oversleeping, avoiding anything associated with exercise and healthy living, and searching for solace in a carton of ice cream.

Authoritarian parents threaten and punish their children, producing short-term compliance but long-term rebellion, distress, and avoidance. Similarly, taking a harsh and critical stance toward oneself may generate some movement, but over the long haul it typically backfires. A compassionate parent encourages the child to learn from mistakes, to constantly improve and grow. These lessons are all delivered in the context of understanding and unconditional acceptance. The child does not have to earn love or work to demonstrate his innate value. Self-compassion involves a similar stance, balancing self-acceptance with committed change and action. Children of compassionate parents are willing to seek challenges and take risks. They tend to be resilient, curious, and engaged. Similarly, you may find yourself lighter and freer, and more willing and able to pursue your values, if you take a self-compassionate stance.

Sometimes people worry that, even if being critical has its downside, being compassionate will lead to complete inaction and sloth. This is an understandable fear for those of us who have continually criticized ourselves as a form of motivation. We have never had the opportunity to try out compassion and see whether, in fact, we do stop doing anything. Given the negative consequences of the continual self-criticism, doesn't it seem worth trying another way? If you find that you truly do stop accomplishing anything when you practice compassion toward yourself, you'll certainly be able to pick up criticism again easily.

> *If you find that self-compassion makes you lazy, don't worry: we humans find it amazingly easy to start criticizing ourselves again.*

EXERCISE **Is self-criticism motivating?**

Do you try to criticize, cajole, and bully yourself into certain behaviors and activities? Spend some time mindfully monitoring your stance toward yourself, emotions, and behavior. Notice what feelings come up when you are critical versus compassionate. Notice whether you feel resentful or satisfied when engaging in actions prompted by threats versus values. Do you fear that if you are compassionate you will no longer be motivated to do anything? Try being compassionate toward yourself for a day and see if you truly do stop working hard or trying things.

Believing Self-Compassion Is Selfish

Sophia is a shining beacon of hope and care in her community. She is the volunteer coordinator at the local soup kitchen, where she helps prepare and distribute hot meals to homeless citizens. She also prepares and delivers meals to sick and homebound members of her church. Sophia organizes drives aimed at collecting medical supplies and personal care items to be distributed to citizens of Honduras and Guatemala who are in need of assistance. Through the foster grandparent volunteer program Sophia reads to children in Head Start programs throughout the city.

Those who are regularly served and supported by Sophia, and cheered by her presence, would be surprised to learn of her private struggle with anxiety. Although she has made significant strides, Sophia continues to have residual symptoms of posttraumatic stress disorder stemming from a fatal car accident she witnessed 5 years earlier. Sophia's friends and acquaintances would be even more surprised to learn how judgmental she is toward herself. Sophia dismisses her painful emotions as silly, embarrassing, and trivial, particularly in comparison to the suffering experienced by those she serves. She views therapy as self-indulgent and refuses to accept a referral from her physician even when he expresses concern about the potential impact of her disrupted sleep and hyperarousal on her physical health. Sophia also refuses to listen to the mindfulness CDs lent to her by a concerned friend. Sophia cannot justify setting aside time for herself when there are so many people in need of her help and support. Only after a minor car accident, caused by Sophia's drifting off to sleep as she drove some friends home after a long day of volunteering, does she consider the potential importance of self-care.

Sometimes people resist the idea of self-compassion because they view engaging in self-kindness and care as selfish. Cultural forces teach many of us to put the needs of others before our own. Interestingly, there may be some biological basis to this instinct as well. In addition to the fight–flight–freeze response, there is evidence that humans, particularly women, tend (or take care of others) and befriend (affiliate with others) when faced with stress. Psychologist Shelley Taylor hypothesized that stress elicits the hormone oxytocin, which motivates caretaking and social behavior.

Just as it can be both protective (when facing a gunman) and harmful (when facing a boss) to engage in fight–flight–freeze in response to a feared situation, there are both benefits and costs to tending/befriending. Caretaking behaviors may reduce anxiety and strengthen relationships, but if we overextend and exhaust ourselves in the process, our efforts will be compromised. Taking care of ourselves through self-care and self-compassion is a prerequisite to caring for and supporting others. Consider the warning to put the oxygen mask on yourself before your kids should the cabin lose pressure on an airplane flight. While a parent's inclination may be to tend to the needs of the child first, suffering oxygen deprivation will likely undercut the parent's effectiveness.

Believing One's Behavior Doesn't Merit Self-Compassion

The view that self-kindness and care are selfish is closely related to another obstacle to self-compassion—the notion that we don't deserve it. There are two variants to this theme. The first suggests that our personal weakness, poor choices, and bad behavior do not warrant compassion. Many people honestly admit they have purposely done wrong and hurt others. As a result, self-kindness, gentleness, and acceptance are seen as undeserved.

> *Kat recently left her husband, Troy, and their 9-month-old baby to pursue a relationship with Max, the drummer in the house band at the bar where Kat worked as a waitress. She tearfully confessed all of her recent transgressions to her friend and confidante Sadie when she arrived at Sadie's house looking for a place to stay. Kat and Troy's relationship had grown increasingly strained since the birth of their baby, Gina. Kat worried incessantly about her ability to be a good parent and constantly sought reassurance from Troy even for minor decisions like whether she was dressing the baby appropriately for the weather. Kat harbored secret concerns that the fear, boredom, and physical exhaustion she had felt since Gina was born were abnormal responses reflecting her inherent inadequacy as a parent. Kat worried that Troy was repulsed by how fat she was and by the dark circles under her eyes, and she accused him of hooking up with other women. She also obsessed over the seemingly unrelenting financial pressure of supporting a child, and she avoided the daily calls from creditors demanding immediate payment.*
>
> *Troy began to pick up additional shifts at work, and while Kat understood that they needed the money, she grew increasingly lonely and stressed by the demands of her new role. Kat tried attending a "Mommy and Me" playgroup, hoping that it would ease her sense of isolation. But the moment she walked in she knew she was out of place. Most of the women were dressed like they were headed for lunch at the country club, in neatly pressed khakis and button-down shirts. Kat self-consciously tugged at the stained sweatshirt riding up above the waistband of her faded jeans as she searched the group for a potential friend. These women were all so calm, happy, and competent; clearly, she didn't fit in.*

On the way home, Kat stopped at a bar that had a help-wanted sign in the window. She was hired on the spot, and she arranged for a neighbor to watch Gina a few nights a week while both she and Troy worked. Kat couldn't wait to get out of the house, and she enjoyed chatting with her customers since it distracted her from her worries. But soon her main motivation was to see Max. She was immediately attracted to him, and she hastily stuffed her wedding ring into her pocket when he first approached her. Within a week, they were spending a few hours together at Max's apartment each night after work. Kat was wracked with guilt about her failure as a parent and her betrayal of her husband, but Max was like a balm that calmed all her fears and quieted her critical thoughts. A month into the affair, she quit her job without telling Troy so she could spend even more time with Max. Kat felt like a zombie getting up with Gina every morning because she was exhausted and sometimes hung over from the night before. She frequently napped for hours at a time while Gina remained trapped in her playpen with only the television to entertain and comfort her. More than once, Kat woke up abruptly at the sound of a car pulling into the driveway and groggily realized she hadn't fed or changed Gina since the morning.

Soon the anxiety, stress, and guilt of living a secret life became too much for Kat. She scribbled a note telling Troy she was leaving him for good and left it with the babysitter. Not knowing what else to do, Kat rushed to Sadie's house for support.

EXERCISE **Compassion and bad behavior**

What is your reaction to Kat's story? How do you feel about the way she treated Troy and her baby daughter? Do you think Kat has a self-compassionate attitude? What makes you think she does or doesn't? What role might self-compassion play in getting Kat's life back on track?

Kat engaged in a number of behaviors that were selfish and harmful to those around her. Her culpability in betraying Troy and neglecting her baby is undeniable. Kat is completely responsible for her actions and the choices she has made. Does she deserve compassion? Does it seem like she is operating from a self-compassionate standpoint?

Had Kat made different choices, it would be easy to feel compassion for her. Transitioning into the role of parent is extremely challenging, particularly if one has limited personal, social, and financial resources. Most new parents feel overwhelmed, resentful, angry, hopeless, and ashamed at one point or another. Yet not all parents engage in harmful behaviors. Some people may react to this story with the thought that Kat was already being too easy on herself, putting her own needs above others', and the belief that Kat doesn't deserve to engage in self-compassion. In fact, when Sadie started to validate some of Kat's feelings, Kat recoiled in anger, claiming that she was a despicable human being who didn't deserve to be forgiven or understood.

Paradoxically, it may be that Kat's inability to bring compassion to her clear emotions and reactions to parenthood contributed to her troubling behavior. Had Kat been able to accept that all new parents feel insecure and ambivalent about their role at times, honor her body for the miraculous task of carrying and birthing a baby, allow herself time to recover physically, and acknowledge the real stress financial pressures place on couples, she may have been less compelled to behave as she did. If Kat had had self-compassion, perhaps she could have tolerated her painful emotions.

> *People who lack self-compassion often vacillate between self-hatred and self-indulgence.*

She may have been less compelled to search externally for love and validation.

Self-compassion can help Kat make amends and move forward. If Kat operates from the assumption that she is valid and worthy and that all humans are flawed and capable of really screwing up, she may be more willing to acknowledge her mistakes, accept responsibility for her actions, and make choices consistent with her values. In contrast, if Kat feels personally threatened by any less-than-desirable thoughts, emotions, or actions, she will continue to do whatever she can to avoid and escape sadness, anxiety, or guilt. People who lack self-compassion often vacillate between self-hatred and self-indulgence. They cajole and punish

> *Self-compassion can prevent us from engaging in the "bad" behavior for which we then beat ourselves up.*

themselves until they can no longer take it and then seek distraction or escape.

Self-compassion doesn't let us off the hook for behaving badly. It doesn't defend or justify unacceptable or inappropriate behavior. Instead, self-compassion, or the understanding that we are imperfect beings, allows us to own our mistakes and engage in reparation.

EXERCISE **The defensive mind**

Take a moment and think about an issue you struggle with or some-thing you don't like about yourself (e.g., "I sometimes gossip about others"). Now, come up with an extreme self-statement about the issue or behavior (e.g., "I am the worst gossip in the world, I cannot be trusted with a secret, and I relish the attention that comes with talking about others' misfortune"). Repeat the extreme statements a few times and see how your mind reacts.

Often, unless we are being mindful, our mind will react by defend-ing itself (e.g., "Now hold on a minute; I am not that bad"). Extremely negative self-thoughts can prompt defensive responses or even excuses, particularly when we are fused with our thoughts.

The mind works the other way as well. Think of an attribute you admire in yourself (e.g., "I am a good friend"). Once again, pump up the volume (e.g., "I am the kindest, most generous, most perfect friend anyone could have"). Often our minds respond negatively as we strive for moderation (e.g., "Well, actually, you are a pretty good friend, but what about that gossip problem?").

As an aside, it can be useful to try to defuse from both extreme statements, positive and negative. You may find that as you observe each thought with curiosity, the emotional rebound of your mind is less intense. When you make room for extreme thoughts, you are less compelled to react to them.

EXERCISE **Your personal experience with compassion**

Self-compassion starts with the assumption that all humans are valu-able and worthy regardless of their physical characteristics or achieve-ments. Yet we are bombarded with contradictory messages. Parents, teachers, bosses, friends, the media, and society at large teach us that women should be thin yet shapely, that men should be tall and muscular, that an A is the only acceptable grade, that one needs to make the all-star team and be easygoing, upbeat, and friendly to be acceptable as a human being. As you practice mindfulness following the script below, take a moment to consider the personal messages you've received throughout your life about your own self-worth. Did anyone suggest, subtly or obviously, that it was contingent on your appearance or achievements? This next exercise can be downloaded from the book website.

Beginning by noticing the way you are sitting. Noticing where your body touches the chair or floor. Then gently bringing your awareness to your breath. Noticing where you feel it in your body. Noticing the sensations as you inhale and exhale.

As your awareness settles on this moment, allowing thoughts and memories to arise that relate to messages you have received about your self-worth. Picturing yourself in different situations and relationships, noticing what you observed, what you were told, how you were treated.

Attending to the sensations in your body, any tightness or tension, and acknowledging the thoughts as they pass through your mind. Observing your emotions as they arise and unfold over time.

Noticing any judgments you may have, or urges to push painful thoughts away.

Just noticing your experience and bringing a sense of curiousness and compassion to what you are experiencing. Staying with any thoughts and images that pull your attention and observing them just as they are. Noticing yourself as the observer of all that you have been taught or told. And bringing compassion to yourself for experiencing these thoughts, images, and emotions.

When you are ready, bringing your awareness again to your breath and the present moment before you open your eyes.

Many people struggle with mindfulness because they don't feel worthy of self-compassion based on their learning and past experiences. Perhaps you're ambivalent about your worthiness. Some days or in certain situations you feel compassionate toward yourself, and other times you don't. Maybe you can understand and comfort yourself for feeling sad over the death of a loved one, but it's not acceptable to feel sad if you aren't invited to join your coworkers for lunch. Having doubts or contradictory thoughts about the idea of self-compassion is pretty common. You're not required to feel worthy or valuable to bring compassion to yourself. What is required is willingness and intent. You can bring all the skills you have been introduced to in this book in response to the thought "I do not deserve self-compassion." Instead of buying the content of that thought, you might observe it, allow it to be present, and bring compassion to it: "Of course I have these thoughts and feelings. This idea of low self-worth is deeply ingrained in me." And you can choose to engage in valued actions in the presence of that thought. You can think, "I don't deserve to be treated kindly" and still treat yourself with kindness. Just like willingness, self-compassion is a stance that we assume. We don't need to feel self-compassionate or have the thought that compassion is the answer. Every reader has what he or she needs to bring an attitude of self-compassion to this very moment. It may be challenging and require some intention and practice, but we all have this capacity. What is needed is a leap of faith.

> *Self-compassion requires only willingness. You don't have to feel worthy.*

Strategies Aimed Directly at Cultivating Self-Compassion

Throughout the book, we've presented information that we hope will help you cultivate self-compassion. We find that often just reminding ourselves that our reactions are human and understandable can help us feel more compassion toward ourselves. When we can see that our emotions are muddy and understand why this is, often we can be gentle with ourselves no matter how intense those reactions are. Practicing a whole range of mindfulness exercises can also help cultivate self-compassion. In particular, we find that the "inviting a difficulty in" exercise can help us soften toward our experience and bring an attitude of kindness toward ourselves. The exercise below can also help cultivate compassion when our thoughts are particularly critical.

EXERCISE **Mindful observation of self-critical thoughts**

This is an exercise you might try when you notice you are being harsh or critical toward yourself. You can also download a recording of the exercise from the book website.

Beginning by noticing the way you are sitting. Noticing where your body touches the chair or floor. Then gently bringing your awareness to your breath. Noticing where you feel it in your body. Noticing the sensations as you inhale and exhale. You may feel the breath in your belly, your chest, the back of your throat, or your nostrils. Just allowing your awareness to settle there for a moment as you feel yourself breathe.

As your awareness settles on this moment, bringing your attention to the self-critical thoughts you are having. And as best you can, observing them for a moment either as words on leaves floating down a stream or as words projected on a movie screen. Although you may feel a pull to judge those thoughts, change their content, or push them away, as best you can just acknowledging their presence and allowing them to be as they are.

Now see if you can associate these harsh and critical thoughts with a source. Perhaps these hurtful words come from an ex. Maybe a friend said them to you in anger. Or you heard it from the popular kids back when you were in school. Maybe this is a message that came from your parents.

See if you can "hear" these thoughts in different voices. Your boss complaining about your performance. Your mother arguing with you about your weight. Instead of perceiving these thoughts as a part of your character, see if you can observe them as the complaints or insults of others. You

might even visualize the messengers dispensing their poisonous messages. For a few moments, taking a curious and
observing stance, watching your thoughts pulling for your
attention like advertisers on a television program competing with each other for your attention and trying to convince
you of the veracity of their message. Each thought tugging
at you and vying for attention like a room full of needy tod-
dlers.

And when you are ready, bringing your attention back
to the breath and opening your eyes.

Sometimes, although we struggle to bring compassion to ourselves,
we may treat others with more kindness or forgiveness, such as a friend,
a sibling, a partner, a child, or even a cherished pet. Although it may
seem awkward at first, it can help to draw on some of these relationships
when responding to your own thoughts, emotions, or sensations.

> Georgia has a strong, loving relationship with her younger sister,
> Maya. When Maya beats herself up for something she has done,
> Georgia typically responds in a kind, loving, and patient manner.
> For example, Maya called Georgia, desperate and tearful, afraid
> that her husband, Derek, might be cheating on her. She was looking
> for clues and trying to prevent a breakup. Maya confessed she felt
> weak and dependent. She wished she could remain cool and aloof
> and hard to get to make Derek want to pursue her. With shame
> and embarrassment Maya admitted to Georgia that she was using
> Derek's password to sign on to his e-mail and Facebook accounts,
> looking for evidence of his infidelity.
>
> Georgia first validated Maya's experience: "Of course you
> want to be loved by someone and feel special. We all want to con-
> nect with someone and have those strong bonds. Wanting that for
> yourself doesn't mean you are weak or dependent on men." Even
> though Georgia didn't agree with her sister's actions, she didn't take
> them to reflect some fatal flaw in her sister's character. In a loving
> and accepting way, she helped Maya see her mistakes and encour-
> aged her to address them moving forward: "You're right that sign-
> ing on to his Facebook account and reading his e-mail were both

breaches of trust. Whether or not he is cheating on you, that's not the kind of person you want to be. It's natural to fear the loss of this relationship and to want to prevent it, yet you can't control his behavior if he really does want to break up. If you engage in desperate actions, it's likely just to make you feel worse about yourself. Focus instead on what you can control and the kind of person you want to be. What do you want to say to Derek?"

Unfortunately, when it came to her own experiences and behavior, Georgia was much harsher and less forgiving. We asked her to imagine that she was responding to Maya whenever she noticed a critical or judgmental self-reaction—to talk to herself the way she might talk to her sister. Although Georgia found this method clumsy at first, over time she was able to develop new ways of responding to herself.

If you're anything like us, you might be thinking, "Well, sometimes I'm compassionate toward others, but other times I can be sort of nasty, petty, and critical toward them as well." Welcome to the human race. It's not uncommon for us to be as judgmental and critical toward others (at least toward some people or at least some of the time) as we are toward ourselves. You may find that as you develop a more expansive and compassionate stance toward yourself, your tolerance for the foibles of other humans increases as well. The point is that you don't need to be Mother Teresa to achieve self-compassion. Model your self-reactions on times when you've been caring to and understanding of others. Or use a role-model relationship to guide you. The images you use should be personally relevant and workable for you. You might draw on the parenting behavior of a fictional character from your favorite novel, the kindness you've seen a friend show his partner, the effective and inspirational way a boss relates to her employees, or even draw from your idea of the relationship between an important religious figure and his or her followers. Whatever works for you.

Developing a self-compassionate stance is both extremely complicated and deceptively simple. It is complicated for all of the reasons described in this chapter. So many of our learning experiences reinforce the idea that self-worth needs to be earned, that harsh, relentless criticism builds character and motivates us to succeed. And yet the solution seems to involve just a simple leap of faith. As we invited you to drop the rope in your tug-of-war with the monster or anxiety, we invite you now to consider letting go of the struggle to prove that you are worthy of compassion. Instead, we ask you to work from the assumption that ever since the moment you were born you have been a person worthy of love, acceptance, and compassion. You didn't have to prove your worth as an infant, and you don't need to prove it now. Instead, the assumption is that all humans deserve compassion. There is no doubt that we all make mistakes, sometimes extremely harmful ones. Yet if we are compassionate, and we allow ourselves to feel the emotions humans feel and make the mistakes humans make, we also have the power to make small and large contributions to our friends, families, coworkers, and communities. Imagine if rather than focusing all your energy on proving your worth you were free to focus on fully living your life.

Of course, intending to practice self-compassion doesn't mean we will feel self-compassion all the time. This aspect of mindfulness is just like mindfulness itself—a process that we have to turn our attention to, again and again and again. We will all judge and criticize ourselves, reflexively, no matter how much we cultivate self-compassion. But each moment offers a new opportunity. When you notice that judgments and noncompassionate reactions arise, you have taken the important first step of bringing awareness to the kinds of reactions you are having to your experiences. Next, see if you can bring compassion to yourself for having that struggle. And if you find yourself instead judging your lack of self-compassion (as we all do at times), see if you can have compassion for yourself for that. And if, instead, you judge yourself for your judging, see if you can have compassion for *that*. And so on. At any moment, we can interrupt this cycle of self-criticism and feel for our own humanness and how we naturally respond to challenges in ways that can make things harder at times. Sometimes it will take much longer than others for us to make this shift, and that's part of being human too. See what you discover when you begin to add self-compassion to moments of difficulty in your own life. Notice how this is possible, even at the moments it seems the most impossible. For us, this is part of a lifelong journey of growth and discovery.

13

staying open when the going gets tough

The exploration and growth associated with a mindful approach to life is a lifelong process. As we revisit these principles throughout our own lives, we constantly find new ways to turn toward our emotions, let go of the struggle to avoid distress, and live our lives more fully and meaningfully. We hope you will too. Anxiety and fear are natural emotional states that will ebb and flow as you courageously face challenges, opening yourself up to opportunities and risks. Just as we—and you— can hope to make mindful discoveries along the way, we'll encounter difficult times that will bring up urges to avoid, withdraw, and shut down. At these times you may find as we have, over and over again, that you lose the mindful way of being and need to reconnect. This chapter offers some of our ideas for keeping this way of being alive in your life even when the going gets tough.

If you are just reading the book through for the first time, we think (as mentioned in the Introduction) it can be extremely helpful to revisit certain chapters so you can more fully apply the concepts that seem most likely to pave your way through anxiety. This may be the right moment to go back and read over previous chapters if you feel like you're still struggling with willingness (Chapters 8 and 9) or muddy emotions (Chapters 6, 7, and 12). Sometimes willingness is more accessible when we have more clearly identified what matters most to us, so that we can vividly imagine the mountain ahead of us as we wade through the swamp, occasionally stumbling and getting mud on our faces; Chapters 10 and 11 may be worth revisiting to further clarify your values.

If you haven't started a regular mindfulness practice or gone through all of the exercises, working through the exercises and practices in each chapter can be a concrete way to start bringing the book into your life. Or you may feel ready to think about what you've learned and how you might maintain and continue the path of growth you have begun. If so, please read on!

Elena had been practicing mindfulness for 8 weeks. She set aside time each morning to do a formal mindfulness practice, either noticing her breath or listening to sounds, and she tried to bring gentle awareness to her experience throughout her day. She enjoyed the time she set aside during the morning, although often her mind was racing with things she had to do during the day, so it was hard to shift her awareness back to her breath or the sounds around her. She found herself judging herself for being "bad" at mindfulness but remembered to practice compassion and that it was natural to find it hard to slow her busy mind. She found that this practice helped her start her day feeling less caught in her anxiety and stress than she used to, yet she still found anxious sensations and thoughts arising as she made her way through the day.

One day she had a presentation to do at work. During her morning practice, her mind kept drifting to the topic of the presentation, rehearsing what she would say, anticipating questions people would ask. Each time she noticed this, she gently guided her awareness back to her breath, imagining her attention was like a puppy being paper-trained, requiring gentle guidance back to the paper each time it wandered off. As she took the subway to work, she was aware of all the anxious thoughts she was having, as well as the sensations of tightness in her chest and the dryness in her throat in anticipation of the presentation. Although judgments of these reactions arose for her, along with thoughts that she shouldn't be having these reactions anymore because of her mindfulness practice, she was able to bring compassion to her experience and recognize that these were human responses to doing something that was important to her. As she stood in front of her coworkers, she began to feel light-headed and faint. Familiar habits set in, and her attention became narrowed onto her physical sensations of anxiety. Elena judged these sensations to be dangerous, and she tried to prevent them from increasing. She had trouble remembering what she was trying to say and had to search through her notes to find her place. Her hands were shaking, and she could feel her face becoming flushed. As familiar critical thoughts arose ("I look like an idiot," "They're all wondering why I have this position if I can't put together a coherent sentence," "I'll never get through this") she was able to notice that these were just thoughts and that she didn't have to get entangled in them. Elena took a breath and allowed her attention to expand. She compassionately acknowledged the presence of anxiety, reminded herself that she had information she really wanted to share with her coworkers, and focused on this value-based action.

After Elena successfully made her way through the presentation, she felt depleted but pleased with her accomplishment. However, when a coworker asked her if she wanted to go to lunch, she immediately declined without thinking about it. After the coworker left, she remembered her intention to increase her social interactions at work because she valued human connection and was missing it. She began to criticize herself for missing an opportunity to take a valued action and again remembered to practice self-compassion and recognize that instinctively avoiding is a natural response, particularly when feeling depleted. She took a few minutes to practice the 3-minute breathing space at her desk and then mindfully ate her sandwich before she turned her attention back to her tasks for the day. She made a commitment to ask her coworker to lunch the following day instead.

The course of change is different for all of us, and you could be at a number of different points in the process, depending on your personal learning history and relationship with anxiety and other emotions, the current stresses or supports in your life, and how much time you've applied to the exercises and practices in the book. You may have only begun to notice a slight shift in your habitual, anxious ways of responding to life, like Elena. Please don't think that means something is wrong. As we've noted before, anxious and avoidant habits take a long time to develop and establish, and living a mindful, engaged life is a process, not a goal. If you've been struggling with anxiety for a long time, this is just the beginning of a fulfilling and meaningful journey. The absence of dramatic change in your life at this minute does not mean you won't experience substantial changes as you go forward. Elena has begun to disrupt her habitual ways of responding and to experience more flexibility. As she continues to practice and apply her newly learned skills, these changes will expand and become even more noticeable. On the other hand, if your life is particularly challenging at the moment, you may find even the slightest change very encouraging, and you may see more dramatic changes as life continues to unfold. Or you may have realized while reading this book that you would like some outside help in applying these principles to your life. A therapist can be very helpful as we try to change long-standing habits of responding (see our suggestions in the Introduction for how to find a therapist).

> *Jin had been practicing mindfulness both formally and informally for several weeks, as well as engaging in valued actions in many areas of his life. Before he began practicing, he had tried to keep his emotions at bay and restricted his life in ways that were ultimately unsatisfying. During that time, he experienced a constant low level of tension and anxiety as he tried to keep things "under control." Since beginning his regular mindfulness practice and practicing turning toward, rather than away from, his internal experience, Jin realized how constrained his life was. He noticed feelings of loneliness and a desire to make a significant emotional connection with someone, so he began online dating. By being mindful during his team meetings, he noticed that he often had ideas to share, but kept quiet for fear his ideas would be rejected. He began to share these ideas during meetings. Jin felt satisfied with his new engagement in life, although he did find that he experienced more intense anxiety just before dates or when he first began to speak in a meeting. He was able to see this anxiety as part of engaging in a full life. Each time it arose, he practiced mindfulness and found that his anxiety decreased over time when he stayed present in a given situation.*

Perhaps, like Jin, you've made some major changes in your life, moving forward where you used to avoid, taking actions consistent with your values. Don't be surprised if you sometimes seem more anxious than you did before, when your life was more constrained. Fully engaging in life in new ways is unsettling, even if it is ultimately rewarding. We hope the mindfulness skills you have been developing can help you see this discomfort and anxiety as something that will rise and fall, not a permanent state of being or a sign that something is wrong.

Some people notice more dramatic changes right away and feel like they're in a new, exciting place, which makes them hope these changes last so that the struggles of the past are behind them. Suzanne found that after many weeks of mindfulness practice, values clarification, and engaging in valued actions, she rarely experienced the social anxiety that had been such a hindrance to her life before. She practiced mindful yoga each day and was able to bring gentle, compassionate awareness to social contexts so that she could interact with people openheartedly, regardless of the self-critical thoughts that sometimes arose. She found her new social connections so satisfying that it was easy for her to continue this new habit of social engagement, which was radically different from her previous actions. She hoped that social anxiety and avoidance were behind her. If you're experiencing something similar, enjoy the present moment *but also* read our thoughts on how to maintain gains when the inevitable challenges arise.

Or you may be someplace in between—hopeful, but worried that these changes won't hold or that you'll forget what you've learned here.

Each of these positions contains hope for the future.

Summing Up What You Have Learned

When our clients prepare to leave therapy, we always take some time to help them sum up what has been most meaningful to them about the work we've done together so they can carry forward the things that have helped them and return to them whenever times get tough. The general principles we've examined together are listed below. Read them over and think about the ways that each was specifically meaningful to you. There may be particular metaphors (like the swamp metaphor, or the idea of paddling out to catch a big wave), mindfulness exercises, phrases (like "drop the rope" or "it's already here") that resonated with you. Take some time to jot these in your notebook so you can refer back to them for reminders of what has helped you when you need extra help in the future.

Summary of Principles in This Book

In this book you learned:

- *Techniques to increase your present-moment focus and clarify your awareness, such as:*
  - Self-awareness (monitoring thoughts, sensations, and emotions).
  - Mindfulness (focus on present-moment nonjudgmental observation of your actual experience).
  - Bringing compassion and kindness to your experience, helping to clarify it.

- *How to turn toward your emotions rather than turning away from them or trying to control them:*
  - Emotions and thoughts (positively and negatively evaluated) are part of being human and give us important information.
  - Attempts to control thoughts and feelings can backfire and increase distress, making our emotions "muddy" and harder to understand.
  - Increasing your willingness to experience all thoughts, feelings, and bodily sensations can open you up to more choices in your life.
  - Recognizing thoughts as thoughts and feelings as feelings and observing how they rise and fall, rather than seeing them as the *truth*, can increase our willingness.

- *Making valued choices about your behavior enriches life:*
  - You wrote about what matters to you in relationships, work/school/household management, and self-nourishment and community involvement.
  - You chose to make a commitment to live your life in a certain way.
  - You learned the importance of focusing on values and process, rather than solely on goals and outcomes.
  - You began to choose actions in your daily life rather than reacting to situations and thoughts and feelings.

Awareness, mindfulness, willingness, and value-guided action (or valued action) are all concepts that you can continue to work toward. They are processes, not goals to be met or completed.

Making Mindfulness a Regular Part of Your Life

Throughout this book we've described a number of very different mindfulness exercises, from breathing to imagery to poetry. Not surprisingly, people usually develop favorites. You likely find certain mindfulness exercises helpful and practice them regularly while others just don't seem to fit your experience. We recommend that you stick with those practices that you've found helpful and use them regularly, but also use some of the other practices from time to time. Doing so can help you bring beginner's mind to your practice so that it doesn't become such a rote habit that you stop truly opening up to and noticing the present moment with fresh eyes as part of your practice. A different practice can bring new challenges or observations that can help to keep the process of mindfulness alive. So

> *Every few weeks, try an exercise you haven't done for a while to bring beginner's mind to your practice and further your exploration and growth.*

every couple of weeks, or once a month, try an exercise that you haven't done in a while to see what you discover.

We also recommend certain practices for specific purposes:

- Mindfulness of the breath is an excellent basic, portable practice that you can use both formally and informally and that is always accessible.
- Breathing space (Chapter 11) is a nice variation of this practice that can help you check in when racing from one activity to another or when feeling confused or out of sorts. In both of those exercises the breath can serve as a quick way to anchor you to the present moment.
- Checking in with your body can be extremely helpful in monitoring stress, particularly given the ways that physical tension can muddy emotions. A brief version of mindfulness of physical sensations (Chapter 5) can help you notice when your stress level has increased, and practicing progressive muscle relaxation (Chapter 5) regularly may also help to reduce your general stress level, decreasing muddy responding more broadly.
- When you are confused by your emotional responses or you have a reaction that seems more intense than the situation warrants,

you may find that mindfulness of emotions, or mindfulness of emotions and physical sensations (Chapters 6 and 7, respectively) can help bring clarity.

- When your thoughts are racing, or you feel tangled up in them, we recommend practicing putting your thoughts on clouds, leaves, or a movie screen (as described in Chapter 9). These practices help you develop a sense of thoughts as separate from yourself and help you watch your thoughts come and go rather than feeling compelled to react to them.

- If you find that you are having trouble seeing situations flexibly and that you are bringing the same expectations to each situation, rather than watching what unfolds, practices such as mindfulness of sounds (Chapter 5) or eating a meal mindfully can help you cultivate beginner's mind again so that you can bring this open perspective to circumstances in your life.

- During difficult times or when you're struggling with willingness, we find mindfully reading "The Guest House" (Chapter 9) or practicing "inviting a difficulty in" (Chapter 12) to be particularly useful.

- Finally, the mountain meditation (Chapter 11) can help you connect to your inner strength and stability, even in the midst of uncertainty and change.

Of course, these are just a few of the formal mindfulness practices that are available to you, and we are only offering our experiences with how they may be useful. What is most important is that you reflect on your own experience and consider what has helped you during particular times or circumstances. Take some time now to think about this and write your observations in your notebook so that you can refer to them later when you want to choose an exercise to practice.

At this point, you may have established enough of a habit of mindfulness practice that you have some experience with what works best for you. As illustrated by the people described above, you may be doing formal practice (sitting, walking, yoga, tai chi, or some other form of martial arts) daily or several times a week. You may be practicing informally regularly and doing formal practice less frequently but still regularly. Or you may still be trying to find the right routine for you. If you're having trouble establishing a regular routine, you may want to find some outside support, like a regular yoga class or meditation group or a group of friends to sit with weekly so that you can make mindfulness a regular part of your life. You can also set up cues to keep your informal practice regular, like noticing your breath each time the phone rings, or at red lights, or in the elevator, or when your baby cries, so that you are brought back to the present moment repeatedly during the day. Practicing mindfulness regularly as you transition from one activity to the next can also be helpful (e.g., on the way to work, while walking to a meeting, on your way to pick up your kids). If mindfulness isn't already a regular part of your life, take a few moments now and think about strategies for regular mindfulness practice that you think you can fit into your ongoing daily life and write some ideas in your notebook. Try some out over the next few weeks and then revisit the list if you feel like they haven't been successful. Remember that if you can't make formal practice part of your life right now, you can still bring moments of informal practice to your experience.

Making mindfulness a natural part of your daily routine is an important way to help keep the changes you have made and to continue the process of growth that you have begun while reading this book. Bringing gentle, compassionate, expanded awareness to your life as you live it will help you:

- notice natural tendencies to turn away from emotions and instead turn toward them
- notice muddy emotional responses and clarify them so that you can listen to the information your emotions are giving you, yet make choices about the actions you take
- reduce automatic efforts to control your emotions that end up increasing your distress
- choose valued actions instead of habitual avoidance so that you live a full, meaningful life

For most of us, no matter how much we practice, it's easy to forget and to slip into a cycle of mindlessness. Having a regular routine can help us remember to bring mindfulness to our daily lives. Other reminders can also be helpful. I (L. R.) have objects on my desk at school and artwork both at home and at school that I associate with the practice of mindfulness. Each time I see these items, I'm brought back to the present moment and reminded to bring gentleness and compassion to my aware-ness. These help me keep mindfulness present through busy days when many frustrated responses arise. Reading books about mindfulness can also be helpful. At the end of this book we include a list of books that we and the people with whom we have worked have found helpful. You may want to try some of these, particularly during times when you feel like your mindfulness practice has gotten further away from you for some rea-son. It can also be helpful to return to the audio recordings of exercises available on the book website when your regular mindfulness practice has lapsed. Although having a personal practice without recordings can help you own your practice more fully, listening to a recording can help to recharge your practice when it's slipped away from you.

Staying Aware of Your Triggers and Patterns

While you went through the exercises in this book, you also may have learned some new things about your emotional responses. Through monitoring and bringing mindfulness to your everyday life, you proba-bly noticed that certain situations, thoughts, sensations, or emotions are likely to lead to strong, muddy reactions for you, or that there are cer-tain times when you are particularly likely to avoid rather than engage in your life. You may have become more aware of automatic responses you have to your anxiety—self-criticism, despair, distraction. Take some time now to think about what you have learned that you think will help you moving forward. It can be useful to make a list of these lessons—the perspectives you have gained that help you live a full, meaningful life, the signals you have recognized that indicate that you are being reactive or that your emotions are muddy, and the situations that are particularly likely to lead to an anxious spi-ral (so you may want to practice mindfulness before, during, and/ or after them). Writing these things down now will be help-ful 4, 6, or 10 months from now, when you're trying to remember

> *Writing down your insights about how mindfulness is helping you now will be useful to you months from now when you just can't remember what you learned.*

what you found helpful about this book. In our busy lives, it can be chal-lenging to remember even important insights because so many other things grab our attention.

Staying Connected to Value-Based Living

Living a valued life is also something that we bring our awareness to time and time again. Our old habits of avoiding distress, acting reflexively rather than intentionally, and ignoring what matters most to us can come back during times of busyness or stress. And what matters to us can change over time, so revisiting each domain of living and exploring what is important to us can help us continue to engage in actions that are meaningful and consistent with our values. Setting aside time each week, or every other week, to look over past writing about our values or to reread Chapters 10 and 11 in this book can help you stay connected to what matters most to you so that you can make choices in your daily life that will be satisfying and enriching.

The Natural Ebb and Flow of Changing Our Lives

Research (and life experience) clearly shows that, although significant change is possible in many areas (anxiety, depression, substance use, eating disorders, etc.), we never fully unlearn old habits, and we can expect them to reemerge, particularly during times of stress or change. Although this may seem discouraging, it doesn't have to be. Any time an old habit reemerges, we have the opportunity to revisit all we've learned, reapply the skills developed, and generate change all over again. And changes that we have already made come much more quickly when we revisit them. In fact, if we catch the signs of old habits early, we can get back on track very quickly if we revisit our past learning.

One of the most important lessons about maintaining gains and changes we've made is to actively respond to any signs of old habits returning, rather than despairing over a loss of changes we've made. Research suggests that a *lapse*, such as a recurrence of insomnia, a panic attack, or excessive worry, does not necessarily lead to a *relapse*, or chronic problem. Instead, lapses are a part of the change process. If we see these occurrences as a natural part of an evolving life, and as reminders that we want to revisit the skills we learned and the perspectives we gained so that we can apply this approach again in our new situation, we can make our way back to where we were before the lapse and

> *Mindful acceptance of* lapses *can prevent* relapses.

continue our process of growth. Of course, it's natural to feel discouraged initially if it looks like we've lost gains or "backtracked." Noticing the thoughts and feelings that arise, including the negative self-judgments that are likely to occur, and bringing compassion to ourselves for them will help us move forward and apply our skills to the new context.

Irina had a history of panic attacks, as well as significant fear that another attack would recur, which had significantly limited her life. By engaging in a process of turning toward rather than away from her experiences, expanding her awareness, increasing her willingness, and choosing value-guided actions, she made significant changes in her life. She found that when she could see her panic symptoms as natural bodily responses that would pass in time and could choose not to act on the message of threat these sensations seemed to convey, she began to fear them less and they actually began to decrease in both frequency and intensity. After several months of expanding her life so that she spent more time with friends and loved ones, pursued new challenges at work, and became involved in her community in ways that were important to her, she spent a few months without a single panic attack. Then one day she was late to work and had to skip breakfast and run to catch the bus. As she pushed her way onto the crowded bus, she felt her heart rate increasing and her breath becoming more shallow and rapid. She felt a familiar pang of dread as these symptoms were followed by thoughts about passing out and her inability to escape the situation. These thoughts were followed by dismay at the thought that all her gains had been lost and that she was right back where she had started. She got off at the next stop, felt profound relief to be out of the situation, called in sick to work, and returned home. Over the next several days she experienced several panic attacks, began to restrict her life again, and wondered what to do now that she was back to her old "anxious self."

A good friend of Irina's insisted on bringing over take-out one night and, while they ate their food, the friend asked Irina to tell her about what she had found helpful in the past for her symptoms of panic. Although Irina was reluctant to think about the approach she had used because she now doubted its usefulness, she began to tell her friend the things she remembered. As she described the way she had been able to see her panic when she learned about the cycle of anxiety and the way her reactions could turn clear emotions muddy and muddy emotions even more muddy, Irina realized that she had grown so used to her anxiety-free existence of the preceding few months that she had forgotten that her meaningful accomplishment had been living a full life, not becoming free of panic attacks. In fact, during the initial months she had continued to have panic attacks but had been able to see them as responses her body had and not signals that she should change her life. In the absence of panic symptoms, she hadn't had the opportunity to practice that response in many weeks, so she had forgotten that skill and reverted to her old habit of avoidance and constriction. She resolved to return to her newly learned habits and reengage in her life. She also began to practice mindfulness in the shower each morning so that she could continue to practice turning toward whatever experiences arose and be better prepared for the occasional symptoms of panic that she might encounter. From that point on, Irina still experienced occasional symptoms of panic, which were more intense and frequent during times of stress or poor self-care, yet she was able to continue to live a fulfilling life and did not experience any recurrences of panic disorder.

It is human to prefer calm to anxiety, happiness to despair, and compassion to anger. No matter how often any of us practice welcoming all of our emotions as "The Guest House" suggests (or how many times some of us write about doing this!), we will all find ourselves attaching to experiences of pleasant emotions and being alarmed by experiences of negative emotion. And sometimes we will compound that response by judging ourselves for the emotions, or the reactions, and/or by restricting our lives. We have spent many years developing these habits, and they will reemerge from time to time. There is no way to keep from having these reactions; all we can do is notice them, be impressed by how persistent these habits are, and gently turn ourselves back to a stance of willingness and acceptance. And we can make this turn at any moment—the moment our negative reaction and tendency to avoid arise, hours after it happens, days or weeks later, or even years later. In any moment, we have the possibility of remembering that this way of being has not worked for us and we would like to revisit a way of being that seemed to open more possibility for us in our lives. Of course, if we remember earlier, the journey back is quicker and easier. But we are all capable of more challenging journeys as well. We just need to take the first steps of noticing and turning toward.

Signs That We May Want to Revisit Mindfulness and Valued Action

The following are some general signs that it may be useful to reconnect to your mindfulness practice and/or value-guided living. You may have also noticed some signals that are more specific to you. In your notebook, write down any of these that you think may apply to you, as well as those specific signs that you have observed in your own life. When these signals occur in your life, find ways to bring regular mindfulness practice back into your life or refresh your ongoing mindfulness practice, explore what matters to you, and begin to intentionally practice value-based action across the domains in your life.

- Feeling an increased level of general anxiety or uneasiness
- Worrying with increased frequency or intensity
- Feeling generally "stressed out" and frazzled
- Feeling checked out or disconnected
- Having muddy emotional responses more frequently and intensely (see indicators on page 136)
- Feeling constrained in your life—like you don't have freedom or flexibility or choice
- Feeling burdened or put upon
- Repeatedly passing up opportunities to socialize or engage in other actions that reflect your values because you are too busy or tired
- Repeatedly engaging in avoidance behaviors such as excessive sleeping, watching TV, surfing the Web, eating junk food
- Repeatedly thinking that things will get better after this one hurdle is passed

When Life Events (Both Pleasant and Unpleasant) Present Challenges

All of us face new challenges in living a mindful, value-guided life as our lives change. Sometimes it comes as a surprise that even positive life events, like committing to a partner, taking a new job, or having children, alter our lives in ways that can lead to increased anxiety, make it hard to live consistently with our values in each domain, and require adjustments. Someone who has been working toward finding a meaningful committed relationship, for example, may imagine that life will be easier once that relationship is formalized. But along with the joy and contentment that a committed relationship can bring, it also requires continual attention and intentional action. Plus, the time devoted to this relationship is likely to lead to changes in other domains of life, like self-nourishment, friendships, or work.

When we encounter life changes, it can be helpful to revisit the principles in this book and redo some of the values writing assignments so we can move forward in enriching and fulfilling ways. Taking the time to re-attend to each area of life, clarifying values in these areas, and choosing new actions that can fit into changed life circumstances can help you stay on course. As we discussed in Chapter 11, the balance across domains may shift and be uneven at times (e.g., if you have a new relationship, you may focus on it so much that your work or friendships suffer for a bit), but over time attending to all domains in a way that is consistent with what is important to you contributes to an overall sense of purpose and well-being.

Similar adjustments take place when a couple has their first child. While this is an enormously meaningful addition to life, aspects of their relationship that used to be easy to maintain may now require some more focused attention and care. More subtle shifts can also

> *Even the positive changes that we desire can throw us off course and require mindfully revisiting our values and the actions we choose to take in the important domains of our lives.*

take place over time (as children enter new developmental periods), so it can be helpful to check in on all of the domains of your life from time to time to make sure that you are living a life you choose, rather than reacting to changing circumstances reflexively.

Changes in our patterns, even when positive, are also likely to disrupt the routines we've developed for mindfulness practice. When I (L. R.) became seriously involved with the man who is now my husband, I was going to my yoga studio five to six times a week. This regular practice helped me bring mindfulness to activities throughout my day. When I began choosing to spend evenings with Josh instead of going to the studio, cultivating a regular practice became more challenging for me. Eventually I began a morning meditation practice (even though I always thought that getting up earlier in the morning would never work for me). Still, each semester when my school schedule changes, it takes me some time to settle into a new routine. Informal practice and reminders are helpful during these times—writing a book on mindfulness has helped a lot. When it is done, I will have to find some new reminders!

Significant, distressing life events can, of course, seriously challenge our intent to live a mindful, value-guided life. When we experience a traumatic event, such as illness or injury (to us or a loved one), when we lose our jobs, or when someone we love dies, our lives are disrupted in significant ways. Or we may experience a number of more minor stressors that increase our overall sense of uneasiness and distress. Pressing financial, emotional, and physical demands need our time and attention. For many of us, these are times when we are most likely to forget what we have learned and revert to old habits—trying to distract ourselves from our pain by eating or drinking too much, working too much, watching TV, or doing other things that may bring some relief in the moment but do not enhance our lives. For instance, I (L. R.) have an overlearned habit of immediately ignoring all I have learned about self-care when my life becomes stressful and chaotic. Needless to say, staying up too late, eating poorly, and failing to exercise rarely help me manage my stress any better, yet it often still takes me a few days to notice that I have fallen into this pattern and may take me even longer to alter it. Sometimes, though, I can remember this habit and begin to focus on self-care as soon as life becomes challenging. This consistently leads me to manage my life much more effectively, no matter how challenging it becomes. The better developed our mindfulness practice is, the more likely we are to notice when we're slipping into old habits.

Sometimes people struggle with the question of how mindfulness can help in the face of such serious stressors. Doubt and skepticism can make it hard to find the time to practice mindfulness when one's life is already overflowing with chores and obligations. And, after all, how can breathing help with financial difficulties or poetry with serious illness? When we work with clients who are grappling with these issues, our first response is sincere empathy and compassion. Life is hard, unfair, and unpredictable, and losses, accidents, injuries, and illnesses bring significant pain. Unfortunately, although what we understandably want is to undo what has been done, the choice we have, at least in a particular moment, is often either to struggle against and muddy clear pain or to be mindful of it. Mindfulness practice cannot directly affect these life-altering events and situations that we so deeply wish to control. But it is a way to be kind and nourishing to ourselves in the face of adversity and to help us bring some clarity to confusing situations and often-unanswerable questions. And if there is some action to be taken, not to undo the event but to respond to it, mindfulness can help us do so thoughtfully and in a way that is consistent with our values.

When someone we love becomes chronically ill or dies, we naturally feel deep sadness and/or fear. Even when we have learned that we can face a range of emotional experiences, such powerful emotions can feel so overwhelming in these situations that we think we cannot possibly withstand them and must try to suppress or avoid our pain. A similar response is common to traumatic experiences, such as an assault or a natural disaster. Yet these emotions cannot be fully suppressed or avoided. We may discover that distraction or avoidance is helpful at times, but we will also learn that we need to honor the pain we feel in some way. A grieving widow may find that going to see a comedy with some friends gives her a needed respite from her sadness, so that she can face it more fully later that night. A sexual abuse survivor may purposely avoid disclosing his experiences to someone who makes insensitive comments about incest or may decline an invitation to see a movie with explicit rape scenes. Nonetheless, the widow and the survivor will discover that there are times when they do need to turn toward the pain they are experiencing, and that they can face even very painful emotions using the skills developed here. Self-compassion and mindfulness are extremely helpful in the face of deep pain; in fact, many people come to these practices only because they have found no other way to respond successfully to this type of pain, while they were able to distract and avoid effectively in response to less intense emotions.

Sometimes losses or traumas provide a context in which it is even easier to live a valued life because they highlight what really matters to us. Death may remind us of the importance of living our lives while we can. When families and loved ones come together in the face of a challenge, all can be reminded of the importance of those relationships and may be able to put petty differences aside or let go of grievances that have been held for too long. Other times, though, when our pain evokes the natural desire to constrict and avoid, these experiences can lead us to feel like there is no point in choosing our actions, or that we should withdraw from connections to avoid more loss in the future. Our efforts to avoid our distress can lead us to be more reactive so that our emotions become muddy and increase the chances that we will engage in actions that we do not choose and may make our lives even more stressful and challenging. Returning to petty differences and engaging in anger at various slights can bring momentary relief and distraction from the depth of our pain, so that we begin to bicker and argue rather than feel sad or scared.

These are all natural responses to loss and pain and may happen to any of us, regardless of how committed we are to living a value-based, mindful life. Yet, again, at any moment we can notice and make a choice to bring open-hearted mindfulness to this situation. We may happen to catch a look of sadness in the eyes of the cousin we are berating for her thoughtlessness, or notice the physical tension throughout our bodies, or see a smiling baby and remember that there are moments of joy even in the face of sorrow. Or we may bring our awareness to our breath as we inhale, exhale, and inhale again. And this moment may stop the spiral, briefly at least, and open up some other possibilities, so that we have flexibility and choice again, even in the face of our pain.

In addition to returning to our mindfulness practice during these times, we may want to revisit what matters to us. Returning to the writing exercises earlier in the book can be a way to reconnect to our lives and our values and to revise them in light of the experience we have just had. Many people who experience traumatic events find that they are able to discover a new or stronger sense of purpose in their lives moving forward, even as they experience distress and despair. Life events may lead to some values diminishing while others emerge, or may change the ways we live our values in particular domains.

Steps to Take During Challenging Times

- *Review notebook and book.* An important first step is refamiliarizing yourself with the aspects of this approach that you found helpful. Review the personal lists you have made. Reread the chapters in the book that cover areas that you feel like you have drifted from. For most people, rereading Chapter 12 will be important—self-compassion is one of the hardest habits to develop, and self-criticism is a habit that often comes back during times of stress.

- *Reestablish or rejuvenate mindfulness practice.* If you have stopped practicing regularly, restarting some type of regular mindfulness practice is an excellent strategy during a challenging time. You may want to revisit audio recordings of exercises to restart your practice and then gradually fade them out of your regular practice. Often, the act of practicing mindfulness will stimulate associations with perspectives you have found helpful and will allow you to begin to experience more flexibility in your life much more rapidly than the first time around. If you have maintained a regular practice, times of challenge provide an excellent opportunity for exploring a different practice for a while to see if new observations emerge. Changing from sitting to moving practice (e.g., walking meditation or yoga) or mindfulness of breath to mindfulness of emotions may be helpful. Or if you think you may be using formal practice to avoid some stressors or challenges in your life that need to be faced directly, you may actually want to reduce or suspend your practice and focus more on informal practice during the challenging time. Although routines can be very helpful in supporting the establishment of new habits, they also increase our risk of operating on automatic pilot. Switching routines can help us bring a fresh perspective to our experience.

- *Practice informal mindfulness.* Challenging circumstances often naturally evoke avoidance so that we are very likely to find that we have become less mindful in our daily lives. In addition, challenges often claim all our attention so that we find it harder to remember to be mindful. Incorporating mindfulness into aspects of our daily life (eating meals, walking to meetings, brushing our teeth, taking a shower) can help counteract these tendencies so we can continue to have the benefit of mindfulness as we face these new challenges. Being mindful in the midst of challenging situations (arguments with a partner, difficult meetings at work) will help us notice our reactions and choose our actions intentionally.

- *Attend to self-care.* Changes in our lives often lead to disruptions in our routines of self-care (sleep cycles, healthy eating, regular exercise, etc). While this is inevitable, we are likely to be more able to respond to challenges skillfully if we put some effort into eating regularly, getting sufficient sleep, and spending some time in nourishing activities. Remember that failures in self-care contribute to muddy emotional responding, which makes it harder to learn from your emotional responses and more likely that distress will feel intense and overwhelming. Even when it seems like there is no time at all for these efforts, a small investment is likely to save you time recovering from reactivity and dealing with values-inconsistent actions you may have taken mindlessly. That is certainly what we find each time we allow our self-care to slip and then force ourselves to make time for it again (and yet we still have to learn the lesson again and again!).

- *Make commitments to value-guided action each day/week.* Over time we all move from planned, valued actions to a more natural process of living according to our values, where we may not explicitly make a commitment each week or monitor our actions but instead hold the concept of living a life we value as sort of a compass that guides our actions. However, during challenging times it can be helpful to revisit this more structured practice and return to intentional behavior consistent with our values so that we do not slip into habitual avoidance or begin to constrain our lives in the face of our stress or pain. We may find that we choose to reduce some of our usual activities or make changes in what we value, as described above. Nonetheless, maintaining our awareness about the choices we are making will help us navigate challenging circumstances in ways that are less depleting and more fulfilling.

Miguel valued providing for his family and took great pride in his ability to financially support his wife and children by working regular hours and overtime at his job. Two years earlier he had moved to a new company with better pay, and his family had enjoyed the new opportunities this increase in salary had provided for them, such as summer camps for the kids and a vacation for Miguel and his wife. However, when Miguel's company downsized, Miguel was one of the first to be let go. The economy was bad all over, so Miguel had to make do with unemployment checks while he continued to search, unsuccessfully, for a new job. Both he and his wife picked up work through temp agencies and subcontracting, and they were able to continue to pay their bills and support themselves, but summer camps and vacations had to be canceled.

At first Miguel had an understandably difficult time adjusting to this change. He felt that he was no longer able to live according to his value of providing for his family, because he could not find a well-paying job to replace the one he had lost. Each time the family had to go without something they had had before, Miguel worried that he was letting them down. He felt anxious about the opportunities his children were losing and his inability to find a job to replace his old one. Miguel found it painful to look at the disappointment on his children's faces and began to spend more time alone in the garage so that his family saw him less and less. When his wife and kids expressed their desire to see him more, he reacted by thinking that this was more evidence of his worthlessness and the ways he was letting them down. His anxiety increased, and he was even more motivated to avoid them.

We can all understand Miguel's response. When we face situations that keep us from providing for the people we love, we all can have thoughts that question our own worth, which may then lead us to overlook the ways we can continue to contribute to their lives despite these obstacles. When the future is uncertain, anxiety, worry, and doubt are natural, expected responses. When Miguel noticed how much he was missing spending time with his family, he began to reengage with them, despite the anxious and painful thoughts and feelings that arose when he was reminded of the losses they were experiencing. One day Miguel was playing catch with his son in the yard, but his mind was caught up in self-critical thoughts and worries. His attention shifted when he noticed the smile on his son's face, and then he purposely brought himself back into the present moment, where he began to feel the peace and happiness of connecting with his son and the simple joy of playing outside on a beautiful spring afternoon. Later that evening, Miguel reflected on what mattered to him. He realized that now that he was working fewer hours he could spend some additional time with his children and his wife, and he committed to mindfully taking some new valued actions in this domain, while still continuing to look for more steady work. He picked his children up from school when he could and began planning family outings that cost little or no money. Miguel was extremely moved by how much the kids seemed to enjoy simply being with him more. When he was first laid off, the kids were understandably upset about losing summer camp and having to cut back, but now they seemed to genuinely appreciate being able to spend more time with their father. Miguel started taking the lead on helping the kids with their homework and starting dinner, tasks that his wife had done in the past. Miguel discovered that he could provide different things for his family—increased shared time and companionship, nurturance, education—that were also valuable and meaningful. These didn't replace the other types of providing he cared about, and he continued to pursue opportunities that might provide his family with financial security. But even in the midst of this new financial stress, Miguel was able to find opportunities to live according to his values.

When lives are chronically stressful and losses are common, rather than occasional occurrences, it can be much harder to find your way to living a valued life. Certainly, some aspects of choice and flexibility are the privilege of economic means and opportunities that regrettably are not available to everyone in our society. These systemic inequalities can make it much more challenging for some people to find flexibility and choice in the face of real barriers and obstacles. Nonetheless, even then, practicing mindfulness and acceptance can help to reduce the fruitless struggle of fighting your own natural emotional responses to these contexts, criticizing yourself, or becoming entangled in your justifiable anger and resentment. Cultivating mindfulness can help you find opportunities to choose your actions so that you bring dignity and meaning to your life regardless of the constraints you face. Viktor Frankl, in *Man's Search for Meaning*, writes eloquently about the opportunities to be compassionate, caring, and human, even in the heartless, inhuman context of a concentration camp. By reducing our struggle with our own responses and clarifying our emotions, we can prepare ourselves better to take action to address injustices and work to change problematic systems.

Whether the challenges we face come from positive or negative life changes, whether they are large in impact or scope, or smaller, and whether they are acute or more chronic, we will all have times when life becomes newly challenging and we need to adjust or refresh our practice and our commitment to living a valued life. The sooner we are able to identify that we are in such a challenging time, the more readily we will be able to begin to implement strategies to help us respond effectively to these challenges.

An Ongoing Practice

We hope you have found some ideas, experiences, or skills in these pages that enhance the quality of your life and your engagement in it as you navigate a mindful way through anxiety. Remember that in any moment, bringing even the slightest amount of compassionate awareness, even if it is only for a split second, can help us be just a little disentangled from our reactions and give us a little bit of space and perspective, a moment of peace or a chance to catch our breath. Even if it doesn't seem to help in the moment, we find again and again that these moments do help over time. And we will keep learning that lesson. Ironically, as I (L. R.) write these sentences, I am sitting in the middle seat of a crowded airplane, hunched over my laptop because the passenger sitting in front of me has reclined all the way back, listening to a child who has been screaming intermittently for 2 hours. I assure you, the first 10 (or 20) thoughts and reactions I had to this situation were far from openhearted, compassionate, or expansive. I notice the tension in my shoulders and the continuous cascade of negative thoughts arising. And I breathe. Again. And gently turn my attention back to the words I am writing and the experience I am hoping to convey. We hope that when you are on a plane, or a bus, or a train, or in a line, feeling anxious, frustrated, sore, or tired, you can also notice your breath for a moment. Maybe you will then also remember why you are going where you're going, or hear a song on your iPod that always makes you smile, or notice the sadness in someone's eyes and feel a moment of compassion. And continue living the life you want to be living, accepting whatever comes, because it's here now.

notes

Introduction: How This Book Will Help You

Page 2: Behavioral and cognitive-behavioral psychotherapy and self-help approaches to treating anxiety problems are, in fact, among the most successful programs in the field of psychology: Barlow, D. H. (2004). *Anxiety and its disorders: The nature and treatment of anxiety and panic.* New York: Guilford Press.

Page 3: Jon Kabat-Zinn and his colleagues at the University of Massachusetts Medical School: Kabat-Zinn, J. (1990). *Full catastrophe living: Using the wisdom of your body and mind to face stress, pain, and illness.* New York: Delta. • Marsha Linehan at the University of Washington: Linehan, M. M. (1993a). *Cognitive-behavioral treatment of borderline personality disorder.* New York: Guilford Press. Linehan, M. (1993b). *Skills training manual for treating borderline personality disorder.* New York: Guilford Press. • Steven Hayes and his colleagues at the University of Nevada at Reno: Hayes, S. C., Strosahl, K. D., & Wilson, K. G. (1999). *Acceptance and commitment therapy: An experiential approach to behavior change.* New York: Guilford Press. • Alan Marlatt at the University of Washington: Witkiewitz, K., Marlatt, G. A., & Walker, D. D. (2005). Mindfulness-based relapse prevention for alcohol use disorders: The meditative tortoise wins the race. *Journal of Cognitive Psychotherapy, 19,* 221–228. • Zindel Segal, Mark Williams, and John Teasdale: Segal, Z. V., Williams, J. M. G., & Teasdale, J. D. (2002). *Mindfulness-based cognitive therapy for depression: A new approach to preventing relapse.* New York: Guilford Press.

Page 5: Given the success of the program in helping clients to both decrease their anxiety and depression and increase their quality of life: Roemer, L., & Orsillo, S.M. (2007). An open trial of an acceptance-based behavior therapy for generalized anxiety disorder. *Behavior Therapy, 38,* 72–85. Roemer, L., & Orsillo, S. M. (2009). *Mindfulness- and acceptance-based behavioral therapies in practice.* New York: Guilford Press. Roemer, L., Orsillo, S. M., & Salters-Pedneault, K. (2008). Efficacy of an acceptance-based behavior therapy for generalized anxiety disorder: Evaluation in a randomized controlled trial. *Journal of Consulting and Clinical Psychology, 76,* 1083–1089.

Page 8: We have found that a mindful approach typically leads to a significant reduction in depressive symptoms as well: Roemer & Orsillo (2007), op. cit. Roemer et al. (2008), op. cit.

Page 8: Research has shown that mindfulness can reduce depressive relapse: Teasdale, J. D., Segal, Z. V., Williams, J. M. G., Ridgeway, V. A., Soulsby, J. M., & Lau, M. A. (2000). Prevention of relapse/recurrence in major depression by mindfulness-based cognitive therapy. *Journal of Consulting and Clinical Psychology, 68,* 615–623. • **effective treatments for depression often include a focus on behavioral engagement:** Martell, C. R., Dimidjian, S., & Herman-Dunn, R. (2010). *Behavioral activation for depression: A clinician's guide.* New York: Guilford Press.

Chapter 1: Understanding Fear and Anxiety

Page 13: the evidence suggests that bringing this new and deepened awareness called *mindfulness* to fear and anxiety ultimately reduces distress and provides new opportunities: Roemer et al. (2008), op. cit.

Page 20: How does anxiety differ from fear: Barlow (2004), op. cit.

Page 20: The parts of our brains that respond to threat react automatically, without involving the parts of our brains involved in deliberation or more complex thought: Ledoux, J. E. (1996). *The emotional brain: The mysterious underpinnings of emotional life.* New York: Simon & Schuster.

Pages 23–24: Our ability to vividly imagine threats also tricks our brains into thinking that these threats are more likely to occur: Gardner, D. (2009). *The science of fear.* New York: Penguin Group.

Page 24: We know there is a future, and we want to control it: Intolerance of uncertainty is a construct that has been linked to worry and generalized anxiety by Dugas, M. J., Freeston. M. H., & Ladouceur, R. (1997). Intolerance of uncertainty and problem orientation in worry. *Cognitive Therapy and Research, 21,* 593–606.

Page 25: The best laid schemes of mice and men, go often askew: This quote is the traditional standard English translation of a line from Robert Burns's poem "To a Mouse, on Turning Up in Her Nest, with the Plough."

Page 25: Worry differs from problem solving in a few subtle but important ways: Borkovec, T. D. (1985). Worry: A potentially valuable concept. *Behavior Research and Therapy, 23,* 481–482. Dugas, M. J., Letarte, H., Rheaume, J., Freeston, M. H., & Ladouceur, R. (1995). Worry and problem solving: Evidence of a specific relationship. *Cognitive Therapy and Research, 19,* 109–120. Pruzinsky, T., & Borkovec, T. D. (1990). Cognitive and personality characteristics of worriers. *Behaviour Research and Therapy, 28,* 507–512.

Page 29: Investigating why people worry has become a focus: Borkovec, T. D., & Roemer, L. (1995). Perceived functions of worry among generalized anxiety disorder subjects: Distraction from more emotionally distressing topics? *Journal of Behavior Therapy and Experimental Psychiatry, 26,* 25–30.

Page 31: What is an anxiety disorder?: The diagnostic criteria for the anxiety disorders are detailed in: American Psychiatric Association. (2000). *Diagnostic and statistical manual of mental disorders* (4th ed., text rev.). Washington, DC: Author.

Chapter 2: How Is Anxiety Getting in Your Way?

Page 46: **Anger and anxiety share so many signs:** There is evidence that although anger and fear are physiologically similar, anger is associated with approach and fear with avoidance. Carver, C., & Harmon-Jones, E. (2009). Anger is an approach-related affect: Evidence and implications. *Psychological Bulletin, 135*(2), 183–204. Also, anger activation seems to interfere with the expression of fear. Foa, E., Riggs, D., Massie, E., & Yarczower, M. (1995). The impact of fear activation and anger on the efficacy of exposure treatment for posttraumatic stress disorder. *Behavior Therapy, 26*(3), 487–499.

Page 55: **This exercise involves freely expressing:** This exercise and the other writing exercises that follow are adapted from acceptance and commitment therapy—Hayes et al. (1999), op. cit. Wilson, K. G., & Murrell, A. R. (2004). Values work in acceptance and commitment therapy. In S. C. Hayes, V. M. Follette, & M. M. Linehan (Eds.), *Mindfulness and acceptance* (pp. 120–151). New York: Guilford Press—and from values affirmation tasks developed in the social psychology literature—McQueen, A., & Klein, W. (2006). Experimental manipulations of self-affirmation: A systematic review. *Self and Identity, 5*(4), 289–354. Pennebaker, J. W. (1997). *Opening up: The healing power of expressing emotion.* New York: Guilford Press.

Chapter 3: Changing Your Relationship with Anxiety

Page 66: **Psychologist Steven Hayes:** Hayes et al. (1999), op. cit.

Page 67: **mindfulness is that it changes our relationship with our internal experiences:** Segal et al. (2002), op. cit.

Page 73: **to develop a plan to work through obstacles to valued living:** Hayes et al. (1999).

Page 73: **developed through our research and clinical work in the areas of anxiety and mindfulness:** Lee, J. K., Orsillo, S. M., Roemer, L., & Allen, L. B. (2010). Distress and avoidance in generalized anxiety disorder: Exploring the relationships with intolerance of uncertainty and worry. *Cognitive Behavior Therapy, 39*, 126–136. Levitt, J. T., Brown, T. A., Orsillo, S. M., & Barlow, D. H. (2004). The effects of acceptance versus suppression of emotion on subjective and psychophysiological response to carbon dioxide challenge in patients with panic disorder. *Behavior Therapy, 35*, 747–766. Orsillo, S. M., & Batten, S. V. (2005). ACT in the treatment of PTSD. *Behavior Modification, 29*, 95–130. Orsillo, S. M., & Roemer, L. (2005). *Acceptance and mindfulness-based approaches to anxiety: Conceptualization and treatment.* New York: Springer. Orsillo, S. M., Roemer, L., & Barlow, D. H. (2003). Integrating acceptance and mindfulness into existing cognitive-behavioral treatment for GAD: A case study. *Cognitive and Behavioral Practice, 10*, 223–230. Plumb, J. C., Orsillo, S. M., & Luterek, J. A. (2004). A preliminary test of the role of experiential avoidance in post-event functioning. *Journal of Behavior Therapy and Experimental Psychiatry, 35*, 245–257. Roemer, L., Lee, J. K., Salters-Pedneault, K., Erisman, S. M., Orsillo, S. M., & Mennin, D. S. (2009). Mindfulness and emotion regulation difficulties in generalized anxiety disorder: Preliminary evidence for independent and overlapping contributions. *Behavior Therapy, 40*, 142–154. Roemer et al. (2008), op. cit. Roemer, L. & Orsillo, S. M. (2002). Expanding our conceptualization of and treatment for generalized anxiety disorder: Integrating mindfulness/acceptance-based approaches with existing cognitive-behavioral models. *Clinical Psychology: Science and Prac-*

tice, 9, 54–68. Roemer & Orsillo (2007), op. cit. Roemer & Orsillo (2009), op. cit. Roemer, L., Salters, K., Raffa, S., & Orsillo, S. M. (2005). Fear and avoidance of internal experiences in GAD: Preliminary tests of a conceptual model. *Cognitive Therapy and Research, 29,* 71–88.

Chapter 4: An Introduction to Mindfulness

Page 78: **But research shows that multitasking is inefficient:** Ophir, E., Nass, C., & Wagner, A. (2009). Cognitive control in media multitaskers. *PNAS Proceedings of the National Academy of Sciences of the United States of America, 106*(37), 15583–15587. Rubinstein, J., Meyer, D., & Evans, J. (2001). Executive control of cognitive processes in task switching. *Journal of Experimental Psychology: Human Perception and Performance, 27*(4), 763–797.

Page 82: **Although mindfulness has become part of our popular culture:** Praissman, S. (2008). Mindfulness-based stress reduction: A literature review and clinician's guide. *Journal of the American Academy of Nurse Practitioners, 20*(4), 212–216. Williams, J. C., & Zylowska, L. (2008). Mindfulness Bibliography: Mindful Awareness Center, UCLS Semel Institute. *marc.ucla.edu/workfiles/ PDFs/MARC_mindfulness_biblio_0609.pdf.*

Page 82: **There is debate in the field as to how much mindfulness:** Although it is not entirely clear how much mindfulness practice is needed to realize the optimal benefit of practice, several studies have found a positive relationship between practice and clinical outcome. Carmody, J., & Baer, R. A. (2008). Relationships between mindfulness practice and levels of mindfulness, medical and psychological symptoms, and well-being in a mindfulness-based stress reduction program. *Journal of Behavioral Medicine, 31,* 23–33. Rosenzweig, S., Greeson, J., Reibel, D., Green, J., Jasser, S., & Beasley, D. (2010). Mindfulness-based stress reduction for chronic pain conditions: Variation in treatment outcomes and role of home meditation practice. *Journal of Psychosomatic Research, 68*(1), 29–36. Vettese, L., Toneatto, T., Stea, J., Nguyen, L., & Wang, J. (2009). Do mindfulness meditation participants do their homework? And does it make a difference? A review of the empirical evidence. *Journal of Cognitive Psychotherapy, 23*(3), 198–225.

Page 83: **Mindfulness Defined:** Mindfulness has been defined in many ways, and we draw our working definition of mindfulness from several sources, most notably Kabat-Zinn, J. (1994). *Wherever you go, there you are: Mindfulness meditation in everyday life.* New York: Hyperion; but also Linehan (1993b), op. cit; and Baer, R. A., & Krietemeyer, J. (2006). Overview of mindfulness- and acceptance-based treatment approaches. In R. A. Baer (Ed.), *Mindfulness-based treatment approaches: Clinician's guide to evidence base and applications* (pp. 3–30). Burlington, MA: Academic Press.

Chapter 5: Developing the Skills of Mindfulness

Pages 97–98: **Research has shown that mindfulness practice can help to decrease: Anxiety:** Roemer & Orsillo (2007), op. cit. Roemer et al. (2008), op. cit. • **Research has shown that mindfulness practice can help to decrease: Insomnia:** Carlson, L., & Garland, S. (2005). Impact of mindfulness-based stress reduction (MBSR) on sleep, mood, stress, and fatigue symptoms in cancer outpatients. *International Journal of Behavioral Medicine, 12*(4), 278–285. Ong, J., Shapiro, S., & Manber, R. (2008). Combining mindfulness meditation with cognitive-behavior therapy for insomnia: A treatment–development study. *Behavior Therapy, 39*(2), 171–182. • **Research has shown that mindfulness practice can help to decrease: Stress:** Carlson, L., Speca, M., Patel, K., & Goodey, E. (2003). Mindfulness-based stress reduction in relation to quality of life, mood, symptoms of stress, and immune parameters in breast and prostate cancer outpatients. *Psychosomatic Medicine, 65*(4), 571–581. Speca, M., Carlson, L., Goodey, E., & Angen, M. (2000). A randomized, wait-list controlled clinical trial: The effect of a mindfulness meditation-based stress reduction program on mood and symptoms of stress in cancer outpatients. *Psychosomatic Medicine, 62*(5), 613–622. • **Research has shown that mindfulness practice can help to decrease: Risk of coronary heart disease:** Edelman, D., Oddone, E., Liebowitz, R., Yancy, W., Olsen, M., Jeffreys, A., et al. (2006). A multidimensional integrative medicine intervention to improve cardiovascular risk. *Journal of General Internal Medicine, 21*(7), 728–734. • **Research has shown that mindfulness practice can help to decrease: Substance use:** Bowen, S., Chawla, N., Collins, S., Witkiewitz, K., Hsu, S., Grow, J., et al. (2009). Mindfulness-based relapse prevention for substance use disorders: A pilot efficacy trial. *Substance Abuse, 30*(4), 295–305. Bowen, S., Witkiewitz, K., Dillworth, T., Chawla, N., Simpson, T., Ostafin, B., et al. (2006). Mindfulness meditation and substance use in an incarcerated population. *Psychology of Addictive Behaviors, 20*(3), 343–347. • **Research has shown that mindfulness practice can help to decrease: Urges to smoke:** Davis, J., Fleming, M., Bonus, K., & Baker, T. (2007). A pilot study on mindfulness-based stress reduction for smokers. *BMC Complementary and Alternative Medicine, 7,* 2. • **Research has shown that mindfulness practice can help to decrease: Relapse into depression:** Teasdale, J. D., Segal, Z. V., Williams, J. M. G., Ridgeway, V. A., Soulsby, J. M., & Lau, M. A. (2000), op. cit. • **Research has shown that mindfulness practice can help to decrease: Chronic pain:** Kingston, J., Chadwick, P., Meron, D., & Skinner, T. (2007). A pilot randomized control trial investigating the effect of mindfulness practice on pain tolerance, psychological well-being, and physiological activity. *Journal of Psychosomatic Research, 62*(3), 297–300. McCracken, L., Gauntlett-Gilbert, J., & Vowles, K. (2007). The role of mindfulness in a contextual cognitive-behavioral analysis of chronic pain-related suffering and disability. *Pain, 131*(1–2), 63–69. Morone, N., Lynch, C., Greco, C., Tindle, H., & Weiner, D. (2008). "I felt like a new person." The effects of mindfulness meditation on older adults with chronic pain: Qualitative narrative analysis of diary entries. *The Journal of Pain, 9*(9), 841–848. • **Research has also shown that mindfulness practice can help to decrease: Symptoms of fibromyalgia:** Kaplan, K., Goldenberg, D., & Galvin-Nadeau, M. (1993). The impact of a meditation-based stress reduction program on fibromyalgia. *General Hospital Psychiatry, 15*(5), 284–289. • **Research has also shown that mindfulness practice can help to improve: Quality of life:** Carlson et al. (2003), op. cit. Roemer & Orsillo (2007), op. cit. Roemer et al. (2008), op. cit. • **Research has also shown that mindfulness practice can help to improve: Relationship satisfaction and closeness:** Carson, J., Carson, K., Gil, K., & Baucom, D. (2004). Mindfulness-based relationship enhancement. *Behavior Therapy, 35*(3), 471–494. Wachs, K., & Cordova, J. (2007). Mindful relating: Exploring mindfulness and emotion repertoires in intimate relationships. *Journal of Marital and Family Therapy, 33*(4), 464–481. • **Research has also shown that mindfulness practice can help to improve: Sexual functioning:** Brotto, L., Basson, R., & Luria, M. (2008). A mindfulness-based group psychoeducational intervention targeting sexual arousal disorder in women. *Journal of Sexual Medicine, 5*(7),

1646–1659 • **Research has also shown that mindfulness practice can help to improve: Attention:** Philipsen, A., Richter, H., Peters, J., Alm, B., Sobanski, E., Colla, M., et al. (2007). Structured group psychotherapy in adults with attention deficit/hyperactivity disorder: Results of an open multicentre study. *Journal of Nervous and Mental Disease, 195*(12), 1013–1019. Tang, Y., Ma, Y., Wang, J., Fan, Y., Feng, S., Lu, Q., et al. (2007). Short-term meditation training improves attention and self-regulation. *PNAS proceedings of the National Academy of Sciences of the United States of America, 104*(43), 17152–17156. • **Research has also shown that mindfulness practice can help to improve: Immune system functioning:** Carlson et al. (2003), op. cit. • **Research has also shown that mindfulness practice can help to improve: Skin clearing among those with psoriasis:** Kabat-Zinn, J., Wheeler, E., Light, T., Skillings, A., Scharf, M., Cropey, T., et al. (2003). Part II: Influence of a mindfulness meditation-based stress reduction intervention on rates of skin clearing in patients with moderate to severe psoriasis undergoing phototherapy (UVB) and photochemo-therapy (PUVA). *Constructivism in the Human Sciences, 8*(2), 85–106. • **Research has also shown that mindfulness practice can help to improve: Diabetes self-management:** Gregg, J., Callaghan, G., Hayes, S., & Glenn-Lawson, J. (2007). Improving diabetes self-management through acceptance, mindfulness, and values: A randomized controlled trial. *Journal of Consulting and Clinical Psychology, 75*(2), 336–343. • **Research has also shown that mindfulness practice can help to improve: Longevity and health among nursing home residents:** Langer, E., Beck, P., Janoff-Bulman, R., & Timko, C. (1984). An exploration of relationships among mindfulness, longevity, and senility. *Academic Psychology Bulletin, 6*(2), 211–226.

Page 99: **Research has demonstrated a correlation between regularly practicing mindfulness and benefiting from it:** Carmody & Baer (2008), op. cit.

Page 105: **we can also shift our breathing on purpose and activate our parasympathetic nervous system:** Bernstein, D. A., Borkovec, T. D., & Hazlett-Stevens, H. (2000). *New directions in progressive relaxation training: A guidebook for helping professionals.* Westport, CT: Praeger.

Page 108: **Mindfulness of Sounds:** Adapted from Segal, Z. V., Williams, J. M. G., & Teasdale, J. D. (2002). *Mindfulness-based cognitive therapy for depression: A new approach to preventing relapse* (p. 196). New York: Guilford Press. Copyright Guilford 2002. Reprinted with permission.

Page 111: **Jamail Yogis's** *Saltwater Buddha:* Yogis, J. (2009). *Saltwater Buddha: A surfer's quest to find Zen on the sea.* Somerville, MA: Wisdom Publications.

Page 114: **from a procedure called** *progressive muscle relaxation:* Bernstein et al. (2000), op. cit.

Page 119: **purposely bringing your attention to an everyday life activity:** Nhat Hanh, T. N. (1992). *Peace is every step: The path of mindfulness in everyday life.* New York: Bantam Books.

Chapter 6: Befriending Your Emotions

Pages 126–127: **Why do we have emotions?** These functions of emotions are adapted from Linehan (1993b), op. cit.

Page 127: **We pay attention to and remember information better when emotions are involved:** Phelps, E. A. (2006). Emotion and cognition: Insights from studies of the human amygdala. *Annual Review of Psychology, 57,* 27–53.

Page 127: **The physical sensations and impulses that accompany our emotional responses prepare us to take action in response to whatever has elicited our** response: Frijda, N. H. (1986). *The emotions.* Cambridge, UK: Cambridge University Press.

Page 129: **Both emotions and physical pain are associated with *action tendencies*:** Frijda (1986), op. cit.

Chapter 7: Using Mindfulness to Clarify Muddy Emotions

Page 136: **rather than being *clear,* or direct responses to the event that has just occurred, they are *muddy*:** Our description of clear versus muddy emotions draws from Leslie Greenberg and Jeremy Safran's description of *primary* and *secondary* emotions, as well as Steven Hayes and colleagues' description of *clean* versus *dirty* emotions. Greenberg, L. S., & Safran, J. D. (1987). *Emotion in psychotherapy.* New York: Guilford Press. Hayes et al. (1999), op. cit.

Page 137: **Not taking care of ourselves:** Marsha Linehan emphasizes the importance of self-care in effectively regulating emotional responses. Linehan (1993b), op. cit.

Page 143: **Anxiety disorders are associated with having negative or catastrophic responses to these feelings of anxiety and worry:** Barlow (2004), op. cit. Schmidt, N. B., Zvolensky, M. J., & Maner, J. K. (2006). Anxiety sensitivity: Prospective prediction of panic attacks and Axis I pathology. *Journal of Psychiatric Research, 40,* 691–699.

Page 143: **people who worry excessively, in ways that interfere with their lives, have learned to worry about worrying and about the potential negative effects of their worry:** Wells, A. (2005). The metacognitive model of GAD: Assessment of meta-worry and relationship with DSM-IV generalized anxiety disorder. *Cognitive Therapy and Research, 29,* 107–121.

Page 144: **Research shows that people can also respond to experiences of anger, sadness, and even happiness with distress and that these reactions are associated with psychological symptoms:** Mennin, D. S., Heimberg, R. G., Turk, C. L., & Fresco, D. M. (2005). Preliminary evidence for an emotion dysregulation model of generalized anxiety disorder. *Behaviour Research and Therapy, 43,* 1281–1310. Roemer et al. (2005), op. cit. Williams, K. E., Chambless, D. L., & Ahrens, A. (1997). Are emotions frightening? An extension of the fear of fear construct. *Behaviour Research and Therapy, 35,* 239–248.

Page 146: **This kind of fusion with our emotional experiences:** Hayes et al. (1999), op. cit.

Page 146: **that we get "hooked" or entangled so that we feel all wrapped up in the emotions we are having, instead of seeing these emotions as rising and falling over the course of our lives:** Pema Chödrön provides this image of being "hooked"; Chris Germer provides the image of being "entangled." Chödrön, P. (2007). *Practicing peace in times of war.* Boston: Shambala. Germer, C. K. (2005). Anxiety disorders: Befriending fear. In C. K. Germer, R. D. Siegel, & P. R. Fulton (Eds.), *Mindfulness and psychotherapy* (pp. 152–172). New York: Guilford Press.

Chapter 8: The Allure and Cost of Trying to Control Your Internal Experience

Page 155: **Imagine if you were hooked up to an extremely sensitive machine:** Exercise adapted from Hayes et al. (1999), op cit.

Page 155: **Interestingly, this inability to control emotions, particularly fear, is actually evolutionarily adaptive:** Ledoux (1996), op. cit.

Page 159: **As Ambrose Redmoon wrote:** This quote is attributed to James Neil Hollingworth, who wrote under the pseudonym Ambrose Redmoon.

Page 159: **trying to control our anxiety when our own experience tells us it isn't working:** The reasons we are attached to control efforts are adapted from Hayes et al. (1999), op. cit.

Page 163: **Although both scientific research and personal experience suggest that attempting to control or suppress anxiety often results:** Wegner, D. M. (2002). *The illusion of conscious will.* Cambridge, MA: MIT Press.

Page 163: **Research with both animals and humans:** Lydersen, T. (1977). Fixed-ratio discrimination: Effects of intermittent reinforcement. *Journal of the Experimental Analysis of Behavior, 28*(3), 203–212. Worsdell, A., Iwata, B., Hanley, G., Thompson, R., & Kahng, S. (2000). Effects of continuous and intermittent reinforcement for problem behavior during functional communication training. *Journal of Applied Behavior Analysis, 33*(2), 167–179.

Page 166: **continuous tug-of-war with a monster:** Metaphor adapted from Hayes et al. (1999), op. cit.

Chapter 9: Acceptance and Willingness

Pages 168–169: **The Guest House:** Barks, C., & Moyne, J. (Trans.). (1997). *The essential Rumi.* San Fransisco: Harper. Copyright 1995 by Coleman Barks. Reprinted by permission.

Page 169: **Acceptance simply refers to letting go of the struggle against the reality of what "is" in a given moment:** The term *acceptance* is discussed by Hayes et al. (1999), op. cit. Linehan (1993a), op. cit. Segal et al. (2002), op. cit.

Page 171: **Willingness Is Not Wanting:** Our description of what willingness is and is not is informed by Hayes et al. (1999), op. cit.

Page 171: **It's as if you're headed for a beautiful mountain:** Swamp metaphor is adapted from Hayes et al. (1999) op. cit.

Page 174: **you just moved into a new house and you:** Metaphor adapted from Hayes et al. (1999), op cit.

Page 177: **Becoming Disentangled from Our Thoughts:** Our understanding of the power and limits of language are informed by Hayes et al. (1999), op. cit.

Page 178: **Complicating the issue of whether our thoughts are true is that statements of truth and opinion are structured in exactly the same way:** Our understanding of this concept is informed by Hayes et al. (1999), op. cit, and Linehan (1993b), op. cit.

Page 183: **Exercise: Labeling thoughts as thoughts:** Exercise adapted from Hayes et al. (1999), op. cit.; Segal et al. (2002), op. cit.

Page 184: **Exercise: Rethinking But:** Exercise adapted from Hayes et al. (1999), op. cit.

Page 184: **Some people find it useful to place each thought on a leaf and watch it flow:** Exercise adapted from Hayes et al. (1999), op. cit.

Chapter 10: Clarifying What Matters to You and Setting a Course for Change

Page 190: **We use the term *values* in a very specific way:** Our work in this area draws from Hayes et al. (1999), op. cit., and Wilson & Murrell (2004), op. cit.

Page 191: **Suppose you really enjoy downhill skiing:** This metaphor is drawn from Hayes et al. (1999), op. cit.

Page 196: **extensive research shows that engaging in actions they used to enjoy improves their satisfaction with their lives and even their moods:** Dimidjian, S. Hollon, S. D., Dobson, K. S., Schmaling, K. B., Kohlenberg, R. J., Addis, M. E., & Jacobson, N. S. (2006). Randomized trial of behavioral activation, cognitive therapy, and antidepressant medication in the acute treatment of adults with major depression. *Journal of Consulting and Clinical Psychology, 74,* 658–670.

Pages 196–198: **Who is driving your bus?** This metaphor is drawn from Hayes et al. (1999), op. cit.

Page 201: **A good indicator that your values are reflections of someone else's rather than your own personal sense of meaning and importance is when they sound like rules or** *should* **statements:** This is similar to the concept of *pliance* from Hayes et al. (1999), op. cit.

Page 208: **The "paddling out" metaphor:** Yogis (2009), op. cit.

Chapter 11: Bringing It All Together

Pages 220–222: **Mountain meditation:** From Kabat-Zinn (1994), op. cit., pp. 136–139. Copyright 1994 by Jon Kabat-Zinn. Reprinted by permission of Hyperion. All rights reserved.

Pages 233–235: **Three-minute breathing space:** Adapted from Segal et al. (2002), op. cit., p. 174). Copyright 2002 by The Guilford Press. Reprinted by permission.

Chapter 12: Overcoming Challenges to Cultivating Self-Compassion

Page 237: **Psychologist Kristen Neff describes self-compassion:** Neff, K. (2003). The development and validation of a scale to measure self-compassion. *Self and Identity, 2,* 223–250.

Page 240: **Exercise: Inviting a difficulty in and working with it through the body:** Adapted from Williams, J. M. G., Teasdale, J. D., Segal, Z. V., & Kabat-Zinn, J. (2007). *The mindful way through depression: Freeing yourself from chronic unhappiness* (pp. 151–152). New York: Guilford Press. Copyright 2007 by The Guilford Press. Reprinted by permission.

Page 243: **the research on self-esteem produces mixed findings:** Crocker, J., & Park, L. E. (2004). The costly pursuit of self-esteem. *Psychological Bulletin, 130,* 392–414.

Pages 243–244: **Interestingly, psychologist Mark Leary recently:** Leary, M. R., Tate, E. B., Adams, C. E., Allen, A. B., & Hancock, J. (2007). Self-compassion and reactions to unpleasant self-relevant events: The implications of treating oneself kindly. *Journal of Personality and Social Psychology, 92,* 887–904.

Page 244: **Similarly, psychologist Kristen Neff found that students high in self-compassion:** Neff, K., Hsieh, Y., & Dejitterat, K. (2005). Self-compassion, achievement goals, and coping with academic failure. *Self and Identity, 4,* 263–287.

Page 245: **wealth of evidence from both animal and learning research that rewarding positive behavior is:** Nakatani, Y., Matsumoto, Y., Mori, Y., Hirashima, D., Nishino, H., Arikawa, K., et al. (2009). Why the carrot is more effective than the stick: Different dynamics of punishment memory and reward memory and its possible biological basis. *Neurobiology of Learning and Memory, 92*(3), 370–380.

Page 246: **Authoritarian parents threaten and punish their children:** Baumrind, D. (1966). Effects of authoritative parental control on child behavior. *Child Development, 37,* 887–907. Baumrind, D. (1968). Authoritarian vs. authoritative parental control. *Adolescence, 3,* 255–272. Steinberg, L. (2001). We know some things: Parent–adolescent relationships in retrospect and prospect. *Journal of Research on Adolescence, 11*(1), 1–19.

Page 248: **Psychologist Shelley Taylor hypothesized:** Taylor, S. (2006). Tend and befriend: Biobehavioral bases of affiliation under stress. *Current Directions in Psychological Science, 15*(6), 273–277.

Page 252: **Exercise: The defensive mind:** Adapted from the mental polarity exercise from Hayes et al. (1999), op. cit.

Chapter 13: Staying Open When the Going Gets Tough

Page 269: **Research (and life experience) clearly shows that, although significant change is possible in many areas (anxiety, depression, substance use, eating disorders, etc.), we never fully unlearn old habits:** See, for example, Brandon, T. H., Vidrine, J. I., & Litvin, E. B. (2007). Relapse and relapse prevention. *Annual Review of Clinical Psychology, 3,* 257–284.

Page 269: **Research suggests that a *lapse,* such as a recurrence of insomnia, a panic attack, or excessive worry, does not necessarily lead to a *relapse,* or chronic problem:** Witkiewitz, K. A., & Marlatt, G. A. (2007), op. cit.

Page 276: **Sometimes losses or traumas provide a context in which it is even easier to live a valued life because they highlight what really matters to us:** Tedeschi, R. G., Park, C. L., & Calhoun, L. G. (Eds.). (1998). *Posttraumatic growth: Positive changes in the aftermath of crisis.* Mahwah, NJ: Erlbaum.

Page 281: **Viktor Frankl, in *Man's Search for Meaning:*** Frankl, V. E. (2006). *Man's search for meaning.* Boston: Beacon Press.

Additional Resources for Anxiety Self-Help, Psychotherapy, and Mindfulness Practice

Page 293: **This list is not exhaustive:** This list was compiled with help from Alice Broussard. Many resources were drawn from Germer, C. K. (2009). *The mindful path to self-compassion: Freeing yourself from destructive thoughts and emotions.* New York: Guilford Press.

additional resources for anxiety self-help, psychotherapy, and mindfulness practice

To support your continued exploration of the principles presented in this book, we provide here a list of resources for help, information, and support for anxiety and related problems, as well as resources available to support your ongoing mindfulness practice, either in connection with a Buddhist tradition or not (e.g., yoga). This list is not exhaustive, and you should pay attention to your clear emotions in determining whether a specific therapist or meditation teacher or yoga class is a good fit for you.

Anxiety

Websites and Associations

United States

Anxiety Disorders Association of America
www.adaa.org

Association for Behavioral and Cognitive Therapies
www.abct.org

National Institute of Mental Health
www.nimh.nih.gov/health/topics/anxiety-disorders

Outside the United States

Anxiety Treatment Australia
www.anxietyaustralia.com.au

Anxiety Disorders Association of Canada
www.anxietycanada.ca

Anxiety UK
[formerly the National Phobics Society]
www.anxietyuk.org.uk

European Association for Behavioural and Cognitive Therapies
eabct.glimworm.com

Books

Antony, Martin, and Norton, Peter. *The Anti-Anxiety Workbook*. Guilford Press, 2009.

Barlow, David H., and Craske, Michelle G. *Mastery of Your Anxiety and Panic: Workbook*. Oxford University Press, 2006.

Brantley, Jeffrey. *Calming Your Anxious Mind: How Mindfulness and Compassion Can Free You from Anxiety, Fear, and Panic*. New Harbinger, 2003.

Forsyth, John, and Eifert, Georg. *The Mindfulness and Acceptance Workbook for Anxiety: A Guide to Breaking Free from Anxiety, Phobias, and Worry Using Acceptance and Commitment Therapy*. New Harbinger, 2007.

Ross, Jerilyn, and Cantor-Cooke, Robin. *One Less Thing to Worry About: Uncommon Wisdom for Coping with Common Anxieties*. Ballantine, 2009.

Rossman, Martin. *Anxiety Relief*. Sounds True, 2006.

Wehrenberg, Margaret. *The 10 Best-Ever Anxiety Management Techniques: Understanding How Your Brain Makes You Anxious and What You Can Do to Change It*. Norton, 2008.

Finding a Therapist
United States and Canada

Anxiety Disorders Association of America
www.adaa.org
"Finding Help—Treatment"

Association for Contextual Behavioral Science
www.contextualpsychology.org

Association for Behavioral and Cognitive Therapies
www.abct.org
"The Public"—"Find a Therapist"—select "Anxiety" specialty

Canadian Register of Health Service Providers in Psychology
www.crhspp.ca
"Finding a CHRPP Psychologist" select "Anxiety" specialty and "Cognitive-behavioural" (theoretical orientation)

Mindfulness
Websites

Be Mindful (UK)
www.bemindful.co.uk
A campaign by the Mental Health Foundation. Includes video interviews with mindfulness students and teachers, as well as links to mindfulness courses in the United Kingdom.

Center for Mindfulness in Medicine, Health Care, and Society
www.umassmed.edu/cfm
Center started by Jon Kabat-Zinn. Includes directory for mindfulness-based stress reduction programs around the world.

Institute for Meditation and Psychotherapy
www.meditationandpsychotherapy.org

Urban Mindfulness
urbanmindfulness.org

Buddhist practice journals: *Tricycle, Shambhala Sun, Buddhadharma*
www.tricycle.com,
www.shambhalasun.com,
www.thebuddhadharma.com

Audiovisual Material

Mindfulness Practices from This Book
www.mindfulwaythroughanxietybook. com
Free audio downloads of many of the exercises in this book.

A Wide Range of Guided Meditations
www.soundstrue.com
We recommend meditations by Tara Brach, Pema Chödrön, Jon Kabat-Zinn, and Sharon Salzberg.

Insight Meditation Talks Available as Free Downloads
www.dharmaseed.org

Zen Buddhist Talks from Boundless Way Zen Teachers Available as Free Downloads
www.boundlesswayzen.org/teishos.htm

Jon Kabat Zinn Mindfulness Meditation CDs
www.mindfulnesscds.com

Pema Chödrön's Guided Meditation and Teachings
www.pemachodrontapes.org

Associations and Retreat Centers

United States

NON-BUDDHIST

Center for Mindfulness in Medicine, Health Care, and Society
55 Lake Avenue North
Worcester, MA 01655
www.umassmed.edu/cfm

Find a yoga studio at
www.yogajournal.com/directory.

VIPASSANA (INSIGHT MEDITATION) TRADITION

Barre Center for Buddhist Studies
149 Lockwood Road
Barre, MA 01005
www.dharma.org/bcbs

Bhavana Society
Route 1, Box 218-3
High View, WV 26808
www.bhavanasociety.org

Cambridge Insight Meditation Center
331 Broadway
Cambridge, MA 02139
www.cimc.info

InsightLA
2633 Lincoln Boulevard, No. 206
Santa Monica, CA 90405-2005
www.insightla.org

Insight Meditation Community of Washington
PO Box 212
Garrett Park, MD 20896
www.imcw.org

Insight Meditation Society
1230 Pleasant Street
Barre, MA 01005
www.dharma.org

Metta Forest Monastery
PO Box 1419
Valley Center, CA 92082
www.watmetta.org

Mid America Dharma
455 East 80th Terrace
Kansas City, MO 64131
www.midamericadharma.org

New York Insight Meditation Center
28 West 27th Street, 10th floor
New York, NY 10001
www.nyimc.org

Spirit Rock Meditation Center
PO Box 909
Woodacre, CA 94973
www.spiritrock.org

ZEN TRADITION

Zen centers throughout the US can be found at
www.americanzenteachers.org.

Blue Cliff Monastery
3 Mindfulness Road
Pine Bush, NY 12566
www.bluecliffmonastery.org

Boundless Way Zen
Centers in Boston, Greenfield, Medford, Newton, and Worcester, Massachusetts; Providence, Rhode Island; Portland, Maine; West Hartford, Connecticut; and Toledo, Ohio. Website includes audio downloads of teachings.
www.boundlesswayzen.org

Deer Park Monastery
2499 Melru Lane
Escondido, CA 92026
www.deerparkmonastery.org

San Francisco Zen Center
300 Page Street
San Francisco, CA 94102
www.sfzc.org

Upaya Zen Center
1404 Cerro Gordo Road
Santa Fe, NM 87501
www.upaya.org

Village Zendo
588 Broadway, Suite 1108
New York, NY 10012-5238
www.villagezendo.org

Zen Center of San Diego
2047 Feldspar Street
San Diego, CA 92109-3551
www.zencentersandiego.org

TIBETAN BUDDHIST TRADITION

Dzogchen Foundation
www.dzogchen.org

Naropa University
2130 Arapahoe Avenue
Boulder, CO 80302
www.naropa.edu

Shambhala Mountain Center
4921 Country Road 68C
Red Feather Lakes, CO 80545
www.shambhalamountain.org

Tenzin Gyatso Institute
PO Box 239
Berne, NY 12023
www.tenzingyatsoinstitute.org

Other centers can be found at
www.shambhala.org.

Canada

Gampo Abbey
Pleasant Bay, Cape Breton
Nova Scotia, BOE 2PO, Canada
www.gampoabbey.org

**Listing of Other Canadian
Meditation Centers**
www.gosit.org/Canada.htm

Europe

NON-BUDDHIST

Centre for Mindfulness Research and Practice
Institute for Medical and Social Care Research
University of Wales
Bangor, LL57 1UT, UK
www.bangor.ac.uk/mindfulness

VIPASSANA (INSIGHT MEDITATION) TRADITION

Gaia House
West Ogwell, Newton Abbot
Devon, TQ12 6EN, UK
www.gaiahouse.co.uk

Kalyana Centre
Glenahoe Castlegregory
County Kerry, Ireland
www.kalyanacentre.com

Meditationszentrum Beatenberg
Waldegg
Beatenberg CH-3803, Switzerland
www.karuna.ch

Seminarhaus Engl
Engl 1
84339 Unterdietfurt
Bavaria, Germany
www.seminarhaus-engl.de

**Listing of Other European
Vipassana Centers**
www.mahasi.eu

ZEN TRADITION

Plum Village Practice Center
13 Martineau
33580 Dieulivol, France
www.plumvillage.org

TIBETAN BUDDHIST TRADITION

Shambhala Europe
Kartäuserwall 20
50678 Köln, Germany
www.shambhala-europe.org

For Shambhala Centers Worldwide
www.shambhala.org/centers

Sanctuary of Enlightened Action
Lerab Ling
34650 Roquerdonde, France
www.lerabling.org (See *www.rigpa.org* for related centers.)

Australia and New Zealand

VIPASSANA (INSIGHT MEDITATION) TRADITION

Santi Forest Monastery
Lot 6 Coalmines Road
Bundanoon, 2578, NSW, Australia
santifm.olg/santi

Bodhinyanarama Monastery
17 Rakau Grove, Stokes Valley
Lower Hutt 5019, New Zealand
www.bodhinyanarama.net.nz

Listings of Other Australian Insight Meditation Centers
www.bswa.org and
www.dharma.org.au

Listing of Other New Zealand Insight Meditation Centers
www.insightmeditation.org.nz

ZEN TRADITION

Listing of Zen Centers in Australia
iriz.hanazono.ac.jp/zen_centers/ centers_data/australi.htm

Listing of Zen Centers in New Zealand
iriz.hanazono.ac.jp/zen_centers/ centers_data/newzeal.htm

TIBETAN BUDDHIST TRADITION

Shambhala Meditation Centre Auckland
35 Scarborough Terrace
Auckland, New Zealand
www.auckland.shambhala.info

Worldwide

Listing of Buddhist Meditation Centers Worldwide
www.buddhanet.info/wbd

Books

Bayda, Ezra. *Zen Heart: Simple Advice for Living with Mindfulness and Compassion.* Shambhala Publications, 2009.

Bayda, Ezra, and Bartok, Josh. *Saying Yes to Life (Even the Hard Parts).* Wisdom Publications, 2005.

Beck, Charlotte Joko. *Everyday Zen: Love and Work.* HarperOne, 1989.

Boccio, Frank Jude. *Mindfulness Yoga: The Awakened Union of Breath, Body, and Mind.* Wisdom Publications, 2004.

Brach, Tara. *Radical Acceptance.* Bantam, 2004.

Chödrön, Pema. *When Things Fall Apart: Heart Advice for Difficult Times.* Shambhala Publications, 2000.

Chödrön, Pema. *The Places that Scare You: A Guide to Fearlessness in Difficult Times.* Shambhala Publications, 2002.

Germer, Christopher. *The Mindful Path to Self-Compassion: Freeing Yourself from Destructive Thoughts and Emotions.* Guilford Press, 2009.

Gunaratana, H. *Mindfulness in Plain English.* Wisdom Publications, 2002.

Jensen, Lin. *Together Under One Roof: Making a Home of the Buddha's Household.* Wisdom Publications, 2008.

Kabat-Zinn, Jon. *Full Catastrophe Living: Using the Wisdom of Your Body and Mind to Face Stress, Pain, and Illness.* Delta, 1990.

Kabat-Zinn, Jon. *Wherever You Go, There You Are: Mindfulness Meditation in Everyday Life.* Hyperion, 1994.

Kabat-Zinn, Myla and Jon. *Everyday Blessings: The Inner Work of Mindful Parenting.* Hyperion, 1997.

Kozak, Arnie. *Wild Chickens and Petty Tyrants: 108 Metaphors for Mindfulness.* Wisdom Publications, 2009.

Nhat Hanh, Thich. *The Miracle of Mindfulness.* Beacon Press, 1976.

Nhat Hanh, Thich. *Peace Is Every Step: The Path of Mindfulness in Everyday Life.* Bantam Books, 1992.

Salzberg, Sharon. *Loving Kindness: The Revolutionary Art of Happiness.* Shambhala, 2005.

Salzberg, Sharon. *Faith: Trusting Your Own Deepest Experience.* Riverhead Books, 2002.

Sharples, B. *Meditation and Relaxation in Plain English.* Wisdom Publications, 2006.

Siegel, Daniel J. *The Mindful Brain: Reflection and Attunement in the Cultivation of Well-Being.* Norton, 2007.

Siegel, Ronald. *The Mindfulness Solution: Everyday Practice for Everyday Problems.* Guilford Press, 2010.

Williams, Mark, Teasdale, John, Segal, Zindel, and Kabat-Zinn, Jon. *The Mindful Way through Depression: Freeing Yourself from Chronic Unhappiness.* Guilford Press, 2007.

Resources for Professionals

Bien, Thomas. *Mindful Therapy: A Guide for Therapists and Helping Professionals.* Wisdom Publications, 2006.

Christensen, Andrew, and Jacobson, Neil. *Acceptance and Change in Couples Therapy: A Therapist's Guide to Transforming Relationships.* Norton, 1998.

Dimeff, Linda, and Koerner, Kelly (Eds.). *Dialectical Behavior Therapy in Clinical Practice: Applications Across Disorders and Settings.* Guilford Press, 2007.

Germer, Christopher, and Siegel, Ronald. *Compassion and Wisdom in Psychotherapy.* Guilford Press, forthcoming.

Germer, Christopher, Siegel, Ronald, and Fulton, Paul (Eds.). *Mindfulness and Psychotherapy.* Guilford Press, 2005.

Hayes, Steven, Follette, Victoria, and Linehan, Marsha M. (Eds.). *Mindfulness and Acceptance: Expanding the Cognitive-Behavioral Tradition.* Guilford Press, 2004.

Hayes, Steven, Strosahl, Kirk, and Wilson, Kelly. *Acceptance and Commitment Therapy: An Experiential Approach to Behavior Change.* Guilford Press, 1999.

Linehan, Marsha M. *Cognitive-Behavioral Treatment of Borderline Personality Disorder.* Guilford Press, 1993a.

Linehan, Marsha M. *Skills Training Manual for Treating Borderline Personality Disorder.* Guilford Press, 1993b.

Martell, Christopher, Dimidjian, Sona, and Herman-Dunn, Ruth. *Behavioral Activation for Depression: A Clinician's Guide.* Guilford Press, 2010.

Olendski, Andrew. *Unlimiting Mind: The Radically Experiential Psychology of Buddhism.* Wisdom Publications, 2010.

Roemer, Lizabeth, and Orsillo, Susan. *Mindfulness- and Acceptance-Based Behavioral Therapies in Practice.* Guilford Press, 2009.

Segal, Zindel, Williams, Mark J., and Teasdale, John. *Mindfulness-Based Cognitive Therapy for Depression: A New Approach to Preventing Relapse.* Guilford Press, 2002.

index

about the authors

Susan M. Orsillo, PhD, is Professor of Psychology and Director of Clinical Training at Suffolk University in Boston, and lives in the Boston area with her husband and two children.

Lizabeth Roemer, PhD, is Professor of Psychology at the University of Massachusetts–Boston, and lives in the Boston area with her husband.

Drs. Orsillo and Roemer have written and published extensively about mindfulness, anxiety, and psychotherapy, and have been involved in anxiety disorders research and treatment for over 20 years. They are coauthors of the acclaimed book for professionals *Mindfulness- and Acceptance-Based Behavioral Therapies in Practice*. With funding from the National Institutes of Health, they have spent the last decade developing the treatment approach that is the basis of this book.

Also Available from Guilford

THE MINDFULNESS SOLUTION
Everyday Practices for Everyday Problems
Ronald D. Siegel
356 Pages, 2010, Paperback, ISBN 978-1-60623-294-1

THE MINDFUL PATH TO SELF-COMPASSION
Freeing Yourself from Destructive Thoughts and Emotions
Christopher K. Germer
306 Pages, 2009, Paperback, ISBN 978-1-59385-975-6

THE MINDFUL WAY THROUGH DEPRESSION
Freeing Yourself from Chronic Unhappiness
Mark Williams, John Teasdale, Zindel Segal, and Jon Kabat-Zinn
273 Pages, 2007, Paperback, ISBN 978-1-59385-128-6